the
blame
game

the blame game

HOW TO RECOVER FROM THE WORLD'S OLDEST ADDICTION

DENIS LIAM MURPHY

Post Hill
PRESS

A POST HILL PRESS BOOK

The Blame Game:
How to Recover from the World's Oldest Addiction
© 2023 by Denis Liam Murphy
All Rights Reserved

ISBN: 978-1-63758-754-6
ISBN (eBook): 978-1-63758-755-3

Cover design by Aldren Gamalo
Author photo by Shyrell Tamayao
Styling and brand strategy by Kelly Lundberg
Interior design and composition by Greg Johnson, Textbook Perfect

Post Hill Press
New York • Nashville
posthillpress.com

Published in the United States of America

*Life is a paradox of infinite complexity
and magical simplicity.*

Contents

Acknowledgments ix

Author's Note: Don't Read This xi

Chapter 1: Addicted to Blame 1

Chapter 2: The Victim Cycle 19

Chapter 3: The Control-and-Conquer Approach 37

Chapter 4: The Roots of Our Addiction 61

Chapter 5: Blame Blinkers 78

Chapter 6: Attached to a Label 93

Chapter 7: Creators or Controllers 110

Chapter 8: The Strongest Force in Nature 128

Chapter 9: The Habit of Self-Blame 148

Chapter 10: Uncomfortable Levels of Self-Honesty 167

Chapter 11: Receivers or Foragers? 192

Chapter 12: Fear—Friend or Foe? 206

Chapter 13: Self-Healing Cycle 229

About the Author 254

Acknowledgments

This book has been ten years in the making, and it wouldn't have been possible without the epic team effort that is made up of very unique, amazing, weird, and wonderful individuals. That is why I am starting and finishing this book with a quote from Steve Jobs. Because whether you are aware of it or not, you are one of the crazy ones:

> Here's to the crazy ones. The misfits. The rebels. The troublemakers. The round pegs in the square holes. The ones who see things differently. They're not fond of rules. And they have no respect for the status quo. You can quote them, disagree with them, glorify or vilify them. But the only thing you can't do is ignore them. Because they change things. They push the human race forward. And while some may see them as the crazy ones, we see genius. Because the people who are crazy enough to think they can change the world are the ones who do.

My family is small and consists of my very special mother, stepdad, sister, and two nieces. You, along with my dad who has passed, have been there to love and support me in obvious ways, but also in other ways you will never fully appreciate. I have tears in my eyes as I feel the love in every cell of my body that I have for you all. And just when I think the tears have stopped, they start again as my extended family comes to mind. The Glaser family in California—you have been there from the beginning of my writing journey. I have told you many times how much you have helped me, but again you won't fully appreciate how your love and support has been essential to my personal journey and the completion of this book.

My funny, curious, and creative friends all around the world definitely see things differently. You have encouraged my crazy theories and experiments. You have opened your hearts and homes to enable me to live the life of a traveling hermit as I discover and heal myself. I am in a constant state of awe at your boundless generosity, guidance, and laughter.

I want to give a special thanks to the team at *Talking to Teens* who helped write the final version of the book. In the same breath, I want to thank Helen, Kieran & Elaine, Greg from Copperopolis, Tiffany my co-founder at RoundTable Global, Barry at MGM Studios, and the whole team at Post Hill Press who have been amazing in helping me edit and put together a book I am incredibly proud of offering to the world. Finally, I want to thank every one of my clients who has been crazy enough to venture into the self-healing journey with me. What I offer is not for the faint of heart, and each and every one of you has been an integral part of this book.

This book and the introduction to my philosophy it contains is dedicated to you all.

Thank you and enjoy what you all helped write.

Author's Note:
Don't Read This

Okay, so that title is a little bit of an obvious way to get your attention, but if you are reading then maybe you are more of a rebel than you realize.

This is a warning. A trigger warning if you like. From chapter one, most of what you know to be true in regards to human behavior and how to be happy will be put on the dock for questioning. Everything you have accepted in regards to how humans heal from mental, emotional, and physical pain will also have time in the dock. It is for this reason I say that recovering from the blame addiction you didn't know you had is not for the faint of heart. As one client said after our first session:

> "...it was like getting the best hug in the world and a swift kick to the head at the same time, and I mean that in a good way, extremely powerful!"

And this is potentially how you will feel after the first chapter. Most of my clients on day one look like a deer in headlights as they try and grasp what I am offering as their very foundation is being challenged—the foundation that has not only been holding *them* up all their life, but also *all of their ancestors* for thousands of years.

The harsh reality is: playing the Blame Game has come to permeate every part of society. It has been effortlessly passed down from one generation to another without question for thousands of years. Blame addiction has unknowingly formed the foundation of much literature in the areas of philosophy, self-help, spirituality, religion, motivation, and healing, etc.

This is why everything we have accepted to be true about our ability to self-heal, transform, and reach optimal levels of performance needs to be questioned. Even the unquestionable.

With each reading of this book, you will revolutionize your relationship with blame, victimhood, control, pain, anger, fear, shame, guilt, and regret. Taking this step to honestly heal from your blame addiction is no trivial feat; it is one to be applauded. As you progress on this journey, the rewards will be great. If you have chronic or acute physical pain, you might be astonished to see how it transforms as you gain a deeper understanding of this philosophy. Emotional and mental pain are no different. Regardless of what you have experienced in your life, profound and unexpected transformation can take place at any time with any person.

For thousands of years we have invested in pacification, developing more sophisticated chemicals, concepts, theories, tools, and techniques to help us control and repress our honest feelings. This approach has postponed us from truly and honestly experiencing our genetic potential and what long-term and sustainable healing and transformation feels like.

Author's Note: Don't Read This

I have no philosophical or religious affiliations. I am simply offering something new. That doesn't mean I am offering the truth; it is just an alternative approach to life. Even though I have many success stories detailed throughout the book to back up my claims, I am not looking for your trust, faith, or hope that this will work. We are used to giving our power over to others. My role is to offer you substance behind my claims to demonstrate that you really are a profound and efficient self-healing organism. You will be the one to put into practice what I offer so as to collect your own evidence to see if it works. You will be the one that ultimately heals yourself.

Why should you listen to me or read on? You shouldn't. But if you do, be prepared to take breaks, and reread sections or chapters to make sure you are fully aware of what is being offered, not what your cognitive bias thinks I am saying. There will most likely be times you want to throw the book at the wall. My suggestion is that these times might be the most important time to either read on a little further, or have a highlighter ready and make notes for you to revisit.

The blame-recovery process might feel like a rollercoaster, but like most rebels you can't wait to jump back on to get that feeling you are free and actually living once again. Each chapter will be the part of the ride you have unknowingly been waiting for.

Enjoy the ride as it is: just an offering. And at the end of the day, in a world of infinite complexity, my message is a simple one—The New Murphy's Law: anything you think has gone wrong is here to help you discover who you honestly are.

CHAPTER 1

Addicted to Blame

Our world revolves around blame to a greater extent than most of us realize. We blame our parents for not bringing us up properly, our micromanaging boss for making our job miserable, our gossiping friend for stirring up drama, and those selfish billionaires for hoarding their wealth while others go hungry. We tell ourselves we were late because traffic was terrible, felt irritable because we were sleep-deprived, and failed the exam because our monotoned finance professor didn't teach the material well. Anytime something doesn't go our way, we immediately search for the obvious culprit, scapegoat, or patsy.

When we can't easily fault someone else for our woes, we do what we do best—we blame ourselves. It is our fault life sucks! We conclude we'd be in better shape if we exercised more, have more money if we saved better, and be on a second date right now if we didn't make that one stupid comment.

This cause-and-effect logic feels so natural we don't even notice it happening. These sentiments are reflexive, instinctual, and often made unconsciously—and they are all based in blame.

Blame is present in our history classes, news headlines, and family spats. We can't seem to let anything happen without asking who was at fault. Who started the fight? Who made the accounting error? Who left the back door open for Tigger to run out? We blame leaders for starting wars, companies for polluting rivers, and parents for raising spoiled children. We cast blame every time we tell our friends another aggravating dating story, accuse our parents of sticking their nose where it doesn't belong, or tell someone, "My boss is ruining my life!"

We love playing the Blame Game. When we're not self-blaming, it works a bit like musical chairs. We cast fault whenever anything disappointing happens, and as long as we aren't the one who is left standing holding the blame at the end of the day, we win! We live in a world drenched in blame, and we can't get enough of it. We enter into nearly every type of scenario with our index fingers cocked, ready to point out the latest perpetrator and make sure everyone knows it wasn't our fault.

One common example of playing the Blame Game can be seen when we refer to someone as an "energy vampire." You may have had the experience of dreading a family get-together because you have a parent, uncle, or cousin with the uncanny ability to suck the energy out of you. Or maybe you've met someone at a dinner party whose sole purpose for that evening was seemingly to piss you off. Perhaps you've even had a class with a dull economics professor who had the mysterious ability to drain every ounce of enthusiasm from your entire body.

Addicted to Blame

It feels natural to think others can drain our energy, but the full truth is more nuanced. Most of us have a whole back catalog of stories detailing how others have disappointed, upset, or angered us. The funny thing is, when I ask people to recount one of these stories, they often reexperience these very emotions while retelling it. Meanwhile, the "energy vampire" or "enemy" isn't even in the room. In some cases, the person being described is not even alive anymore. So who is actually draining the storyteller's energy? Who is making them feel disappointed, upset, or angry?

Blame isn't just about finding fault for something we think has gone wrong; it is holding someone responsible for the way we feel. Blame creates attachment to someone else being the reason we feel the way we do. Consider the person you admire most in the world, like a supportive family member, inspiring influencer, or a key figure in history. While you may respect this individual and find them inspirational, others might think they're annoying. If everyone wouldn't universally see this person as a role model, then can you really hold them responsible for annoying or inspiring you? Aren't they simply doing or saying something *you* agree or disagree with? So maybe it is *you* and not *them* that is ultimately responsible for how you feel and your reactions.

It can be uncomfortable, but enlightening, to realize the only person who has an impact on your energy or emotional state is you. You are the one person in the world who ultimately drains your energy, makes you mad, or motivates you. If you are thinking you know this, which is why *you don't let people affect you*, you are still unknowingly playing the Blame Game. You still think it was them that impacted your emotional state and that you can "control" your response, but actually it had nothing to do with them. We can both be watching Donald Trump give a speech, but one of us gets angry and the other is inspired. Same person, same speech, same delivery—two completely different reactions.

Take something as simple as comedy. Do you remember the last joke that had you doubled over in laughter? Was it the joke that made you laugh or the way it was told? This debate can split a room of comedians in two. One half categorically declares that it all comes down to delivery, while the others proclaim writing is everything. But what if the determining factor isn't writing or delivery? If some people find a certain stand-up comic hilarious while others find them offensive, then the answer can't be that the joke or comedian made the audience laugh. The laughter comes from somewhere within the listener. Otherwise we would all like the same comic and material.

Blame has become so infused with our cause-and-effect logic we can't imagine a world without it, especially when it comes to achieving healing and happiness. This is why the path of least resistance is to find a scapegoat for why we think our lives are not going the way we think they should. We often don't need to look much further than our parents or some other family member for the reason we are "messed up." It feels like second nature to search for people or events that we think are the root cause of our problems, not realizing this is a perfect example of the Blame Game in action. Just because we have done something for a long time, or that something feels intuitive or instinctive, doesn't mean it shouldn't be questioned.

Even the most long-standing and progressive philoso-phies, self-help frameworks, and therapeutic approaches are steeped in blame. The stoic way of life recognizes that our per-ceptions determine our thoughts and emotions. This is often illustrated by showing two people standing at either end of the number '6' drawn on the ground—both pointing at it telling each other they are wrong as one sees a '6' and the other '9.' As the poet and naturalist Henry David Thoreau claimed, "It's not what you look at that matters, it's what you see." Many peo-ple interpret this as—change your perception, change your life. But, there is more to the story. There is a profound difference in the outcome if you force your perception to chance or if it changes as a by-product of new awareness.

Probably the most commonly offered solution to change our perception is to force ourselves into a positive mental atti-tude, practice gratitude, forgive and forget, and let go of our anger and fear. Simple. But this approach is unsustainable because it is ultimately steeped in blame: If we aren't happy, it's our own damn fault…. Happiness is a choice…. We just need to control our emotions and responses better. Because we have accepted blame's presence in our lives, there has been lit-tle curiosity to explore or unpack it, meaning its far-reaching impact continues to proliferate unhindered into every aspect of our lives.

Everywhere we turn, we are knowingly and unknowingly encouraging each other to join in and play the Blame Game. Deep down, we know blame isn't the answer. We regularly hear ourselves say, "I know I shouldn't blame, but…" followed by some creative justification. But we all keep doing it. Why? Because blaming has transcended its game status to become an addiction. And what makes this addiction different from all others is that we don't know we all have it, so there has been no attempt at recovery.

We're Hooked on Blame

The harsh reality is that casting blame is satisfying. It's rewarding to receive confirmation we won't get in trouble and that we were right and they were wrong. And if this is followed by an apology, or "I should have listened to you," it can feel like the best hug in the world. Dopamine and endorphins rush through our veins. A surge of righteousness can follow as we confirm, "I told you that would happen." The feeling of being right can be addictive.

If blame has the potential to inflate our status and sense of self-worth, why wouldn't we want that same "high" again? And again? It's harmless, right? It picks us up like a warm cup of coffee. But when does one cup turn into two? When does a glass of wine a night turn into a whole bottle? We justify an extra Starbucks midmorning after a late night finishing a report. We hear ourselves say, "Shall we open another bottle? I deserve it after the day I've had!" But when do our behaviors pass from harmless fun into pain and misery?

Addictions creep up on us gradually. At first, we experiment with a certain behavior occasionally. Before we know it, our cravings become a normal part of our day. We fit in our addiction wherever we can. Early on, the habit is manageable and doesn't have a serious impact on our lives, so we continue. We seek out similar people to make ourselves feel normal. Eventually, we need more to achieve the same feeling.

The fun stops as our mental and physical pain and discomfort increases. It is a process many are familiar with.

Most behaviors cross a threshold, after which we become very aware we are hooked. We try to stop and realize we can't. We notice we're thinking about the behavior obsessively. We can see that our compulsion is affecting the rest of our life. We're aware we are smoking, drinking, eating, or gambling in a way that occupies our thoughts and influences our motivations and health. It is only when our creative justifications no longer work and our health or circumstances become too painful that we start to think about getting help.

This is where our addiction to playing the Blame Game is different from all other addictions. We are unaware of its presence, so we don't fully appreciate its profound impact on our life as well as our mental and physical health. We know we are blaming but we don't realize how reliant we are on it to function. Because blame feels so normal, we have no inclination to start the recovery process. In fact, the Blame Game is so common we think it's an innate part of being human. It has impacted how we perceive the human experience to the point that frustration, anger, and conflict are seen as normal emotional states—when in fact they are the direct consequence of blame, which is a uniquely learnt human trait that isn't found anywhere else in nature.

It has resulted in us buying the biggest myth ever sold: that our mind, body, and soul are doing all they can to keep us in our comfort zone and prevent us from reaching our potential. We think we are constantly malfunctioning like a piece of software, doing all we can to self-sabotage and hold ourselves back. None of this is true.

Most dependencies mature over many years, but the Blame Game has been playing out undetected for many millennia. As a result, we are in the advanced stages of an addiction we don't know we have. And the fact that it is an addiction every human shares goes a long way in explaining why it has gone undetected for so long. So we continue to feed each other's blame addiction without knowing it.

Like other more obvious addictions, our compulsive relationship with blame eventually leads to excessive physical, emotional, and mental pain. It results in feeling fearful, lost, never satisfied, and thinking *Is this it? Is life supposed to be this painful and unfair?* Except, because of the very nature of blame, we effortlessly attribute this pain to other things. Our boss is the reason we lost our job. Our spouse is the reason we are unhappy. We reason that our back hurts because we are sitting all day, but complain that the new standing desk that our colleague raves about has made our back worse. As will become very evident, it isn't our boss, wife, or our colleague's rubbish advice that causes our mental and physical pain—it is our addiction to blame, as this determines what we perceive and think about during these moments.

The effects of our blame addiction are largely invisible because we blame them on a variety of other causes. It is the equivalent of blaming the bar snacks for the reason you're drunk.

If we are chronically gambling, drinking, watching pornography, or using opioids, we know we are engaging in these behaviors too much. The impact is obvious. Our health and relationships show signs of pain and stress. Our loved ones intervene and tell us we have a problem. But this isn't the case when it comes to our blame addiction. Often, we know we are excessively casting blame, but because we see it as a normal human thing to do, we shrug it off. The Blame Game goes on unhindered, and it is happening much more than we realize. As a result, we don't see how we have been feeding our addiction in pretty much every conversation we have.

Blame has become such an accepted part of our lives that we think we already know the simple solution if we do happen to notice it is getting out of hand: we step into our masculine energy and try to force change. Most people who talk about blame tell you—"DON'T blame!" It is the same advice the Happiness Gurus offer when they lament that "happiness is a choice, so drop negative thoughts. Stop torturing yourself. Be grateful, love yourself, and choose positive thoughts and you will be happy." Well, if this approach to changing our lives was sustainable, there wouldn't be any issues or addictions in the world.

This is like telling a sugar addict to stop eating sugar! It doesn't work as a long-term solution. The reason it doesn't work is manifold, but the foundational reason is that it relies on control to achieve success. Controlling anything requires withdrawals from an energy supply that is finite. Meaning controlling any behavior is temporary and so maintains a high level of fear as we brace ourselves for the possible relapse. Even if we manage to sustain the illusion of control for an extended time, often we replace our addictions with more "healthy" alternatives like exercise, the latest diet, meditation, or other mindfulness practices. It feels normal to live this way because our blame addiction has been around for thousands of years. As such, it's similar to how any addict gets more skilled at finding ways to hide, satisfy, and justify their addiction: we have become expert blamers, with countless different ways of getting our "fix." As such, blame is not only imbedded in our everyday language, it is fully interwoven into the very fabric of our corporate and social life.

As I mentioned before, blame's impact is much more far reaching than we are aware of. It often goes unrecognized that every time we play the Blame Game we cast ourselves as victims. It's not a nice feeling or thought to see yourself as a victim, but even with all the self-control in the world, one goes hand in hand with the other. Which is why becoming aware of this victimhood is the first step to healing from the addiction we didn't even know we had.

Blame Leads to a Victim Mindset

As soon as you blame, you instantly become a victim. Stubbed your toe on a chair? Your partner forgot to push it in! And then you ran late to your meeting because you had to address your wounded toe, so your boss chewed you out and you had a totally rotten day, which all started with your selfish partner who couldn't be bothered to take a second to push in the chair. Or you might experience the same situation and choose to cast blame in a different direction. Perhaps you decide the new chair your partner bought was poorly designed or placed in a stupid place and rationalize that any reasonable person would stub their toe on it. Or you may direct the blame inward at yourself for being so careless. Why are you always doing clumsy things like this? Why can't you be more graceful like your sister? There are many possible ways you could take this reasoning. But the basic thought process is the same: the day sucked because it got off to a horrible start when you stubbed your toe. And someone is at fault for that.

Addicted to Blame

Anytime we play the Blame Game, we naturally step into the victim role. While looking for who is at fault, we become a victim of their perceived negligence or malevolence. And that feeling of victimhood is amplified when we blame ourselves for being lazy, stupid, weak, or clumsy or being in the wrong place at the wrong time. Interestingly, even though there are different degrees of victimhood, from being forced from your home due to a war to your plane being delayed, our response is not always proportionate or consistent. Classing ourselves or others as the innocent victim is not as clear-cut as we may think. While one person is feeling the pain of their circumstance, another is starting a business or striking up a new relationship.

When a client is telling me about their troubles with their parents, boss, or partner, they will often be oblivious to the fact they are swimming in blame and feelings of victimhood. Full of justification for the perceived wrongs that have been committed, they will dig their heels in trying to convince me (and themselves) they were the innocent victim in the story. After fifteen years of researching the victim mindset and taking many people through the blame-recovery process, I can confidently say, as complex as these stories seem on the surface due to all the behavioral psychological rabbit holes you can venture down, they all stem from the same simple premise—you think something happened that shouldn't have based on the information, awareness, and wisdom that was available.

Being a victim in life comes with certain connotations, especially when something happens that isn't seen as extreme. This is why when I ask people whether they see themselves as victims, they vehemently deny it. In a world of ultra-positivity and never-give-up Rocky-endorsed motivational rhetoric, being a victim is tantamount to failing at life. When I said to a billionaire client that he was being a victim, he balked at the suggestion. He assured me I was wrong. He spent his day making sure he was anything but a victim. This assurance came after a story where he angrily complained about not being able to enter the first-class lounge before his recent flight. Because we haven't made the connection between blaming and being a victim, we don't realize how often we are in this mindset and the enormous energy it takes to control and deal with the painful side effects that result. It is why—regardless of what wealth, adulation, or beauty you have—it doesn't equate to being happy.

By definition, victims are powerless and often seen as passive and weak. They have no agency. They are blown around helplessly by the winds of hope and fate. In certain situations, seeing yourself as a victim goes against the well-recited mantra that life is about taking the bull by the horns and proving we are winners, not losers.

Even though we typically don't like to be accused of being a victim or admit when we are playing the victim card, we continually seek it out (often without realizing it). If you have ever complained to a friend about feeling obligated to do your mother a favor, you have played the victim. If you've griped about a thoughtless driver who cut you off on the freeway, you were casting yourself in the victim role. And if you've told someone that they must not have been listening because you explained yourself very clearly, then you've made yourself a victim of another person's ineptitude.

You might defend yourself and say you are not blaming or being a victim, you are just stating facts. But are your version of the facts, universal facts? You might be seeing a "6" when someone else is seeing a "9." There is cognitive bias to consider, and if you are angered by the facts you perceive, then we have to revisit the principle above—it is you that makes you angry; it is not the other person and how they behaved. As much as you believe you have logical or moral grounds for such accusations and reactions, this doesn't change the fact that we constantly use blame to make sense of the world, and in doing so we repeatedly become victims.

Anger is only felt in the presence of blame, and saying you are NOT angry, blaming, or being a victim doesn't mean you are not. It is often a way of pushing our honest feelings under the rug, hoping the rug is heavy enough to keep them from revealing themselves. While we are in this denial, we don't realize that our undercurrent of victimhood is influencing our relationships, health and happiness, and every decision. It leads us to create a very different reality to someone who isn't playing the role of victim.

I once overheard a conversation between two women at a cafe in Dubai. One complained about her selfish boyfriend who had not offered to take her out for their one-year anniversary. Her friend, based on the information she was given, sympathetically agreed that the boyfriend was a complete ass. This was just the fuel the first woman needed to call her boyfriend right then and give him the ear bashing he deserved and end the relationship.

But imagine if there was more self-honesty, awareness, and wisdom available. Maybe the women would consider alternative possibilities to the blame and victim narrative. Perhaps the girlfriend had forgotten to mention how insistent she was in telling her boyfriend she didn't want to make it a big thing. Maybe she'd been withdrawing slowly for months in an unconscious effort to push her boyfriend away and this was the perfect opportunity to get her friend's support to justify her breakup.

No matter the case, the act of blaming her boyfriend closed her mind to other possibilities, which fueled her anger and led to her righteous phone call. But just as it isn't an "energy vampire" who sucks our energy, can this woman really blame her boyfriend for causing her anger? The easy blame-based response is yes. This conclusion takes no effort, in the same way an alcoholic decides another drink at the end of an all-day binge is the right choice. No one really knows, including her friend, the details of their relationship. Anything could be happening behind closed doors. The point is, in that moment the girlfriend perceived herself as the victim and him the oppressor because she felt hurt. The challenging question to answer is: Who actually makes us feel hurt?

There is an important reason I focus on helping my clients understand this principle first: that it is their own blame-based perception that makes them feel hurt or angry, not what the other person did or said. Otherwise, they will take their blame addiction and victim mindset into every other relationship. It gets extremely frustrating and exhausting as the honeymoon period in our romantic relationships becomes shorter and the subsequent pain and conflict arrive sooner. Then it isn't long before we enter the final states of our blame addiction and proclaim, "All men are shit!" Or "All women are bitches!"

Our painful patterns don't repeat because of our past experiences; they repeat because we are *blaming* them for being the reason we are not getting what we want. The longer this goes on, the more unhappy we become and the more we look for the advantages that come with being a victim.

Advantages of Being a Victim

We label someone a victim when we believe they had no contribution to the experience. They are the innocent bystander, and life whacked them over the head with a two-by-four for no reason but to confirm *life is unfair*. That is unless the painful experience is accompanied by what the person sees as a reward. Then suddenly it all makes sense and order is restored and they are happy. However, when we think we had no contribution and don't immediately see an obvious benefit, we think we have been treated unfairly and we become unhappy (or ill) as a by-product.

I recently spoke with a woman who was distraught over corruption in a foreign country. Because of the lack of regulation there, she told me, she lost money on an investment. However, three months prior, she'd bragged to me about how the same corruption helped her secure an advantageous deal. The same players were involved in both stories. However, in the latest instance she thought it was unfair, so she perceived herself as the innocent victim and became upset. She became stressed and ill because she really didn't see her contribution. Not only did she reenter a corrupt system, she was full of blame that was directed at a recent boyfriend for leaving her stranded in a foreign country. The more she blamed her ex-boyfriend and business partner, the more of a victim she felt and the more of a victim story she experienced. Her situation became so extreme her family had to step in and finance her plane ticket back home.

The reality is that playing the victim role comes with advantages. The lady above admitted to me she was feeling homesick for many months. She was trying to make it work to prove to friends and family she could do it. But in the meantime, she had run out of money. There is an argument to say being a victim gave her the push to get her to do something she wasn't good at doing—asking her family for help. These events can happen unconsciously. Other times the person is very aware they are playing the victim to their advantage.

You don't have to look much further than a soccer match to see this play out. Acting injured is part and parcel of the players' winning strategy. Some players are better at being thespians than others, but even amateur dramatics can win games. It can be a comical scene when you have one player writhing on the turf doing their best to be seen as the innocent victim while another is standing over them in a state of indignation trying to convince the referee they are the unfortunate bystander. Each is desperately trying to win a victim card and avoid a red card.

The stakes can be high as to whether you are seen as the victim. Pointing our finger at others can help us get an insurance payout or gain custody of our children after a drawn-out court case. When we can successfully convince people we've been wronged, we can often get rewarded. We have an entire legal system based on this victim/villain relationship. A lawyer's ability to turn a villain into a victim and a victim into a villain is why people pay so much for the best in the business. It highlights that not all is as it may seem on the surface. There's often more playing out behind the scenes, but the question is: are you curious enough to take a look?

Addicted to Blame

You could also say that feelings of victimhood have been used to revolutionize corrupt governments. Being pissed off at the system for holding us down can motivate us to seek change. It can often feel righteous and justified to bring blame into the equation, not realizing that maybe it was our blame addiction that got us to the point where we needed a revolution.

As much as there are short-term wins, there are side effects to playing the Blame Game too. Like any game, it can be fun. But even the most enjoyable games become exhausting. Playing the Blame Game for an extended time is energy intensive, and we have been playing for thousands of years. It is easy to believe our physical and mental exhaustion is the result of a long day at work, but is this always the case? What if it is actually because we've been wading through blame all day, looking for ways to implicate others, and trying to avoid being labeled as the cause of the problem? One hour in this state of mind is exhausting, let alone a ten-hour day.

At this point, it might be easy to conclude the Blame Game is messing up our lives. But this makes blame the enemy and just gives us another thing to blame. The goal here is not to blame blame but to establish a new relationship with it.

Once you become aware of the many places blame is present in your life and learn to listen in a unique way, you will notice your behavior naturally changes and your perception of others' behavior changes as well. Your fear of being wrong and need to assert your dominance lessens along with your stress, anger, anxiety, shame, guilt, and regret. Your mind opens to other possibilities as you no longer feel the urge to find something to blame your feelings on. This is the perfect environment for new levels of regeneration and rejuvenation to take place.

I am going to repeat what was in chapter 0 as it is very important to what follows in the rest of the book. Blame has come to permeate every part of society. It has been effortlessly passed down from one generation to another without question for thousands of years. Blame addiction has unknowingly formed the foundation of much literature in the areas of philosophy, self-help, spirituality, religion, motivation, and healing.

This is why everything we have accepted to be true about our ability to self-heal, transform, and reach optimal levels of performance needs to be put in the dock for questioning. Even the unquestionable.

For thousands of years, we have invested in pacification, developing more sophisticated chemicals, concepts, theories, tools, and techniques to help us control and repress our honest feelings. This approach has postponed us from truly and honestly experiencing our genetic potential and what long-term sustainable healing and transformation feels like.

Now that you know you have an addiction to blame you didn't know you had, it is time to unpack the Victim Cycle you didn't know you were in.

CHAPTER 2

The Victim Cycle

When we play the Blame Game, we participate in a basic four-step loop known as the Victim Cycle. First, we resort to blame when we think something doesn't go our way. Next, we become a victim, followed by the third step, fear, or its repackaged name, anxiety. Finally, we seek to control ourselves or the situation. As logical as this final step seems, seeking control keeps us in the loop. Control is temporary, and it isn't long before we find ourselves feeling out of control and casting blame once again.

Let's say you enter the Victim Cycle when you find yourself feeling tired after interacting with a certain friend. Naturally, you blame her. You have told yourself many times she's a negative Nancy! Regardless of how much you pump yourself up, telling yourself you have been friends for a long time, this lethargic feeling happens every time you get together with her.

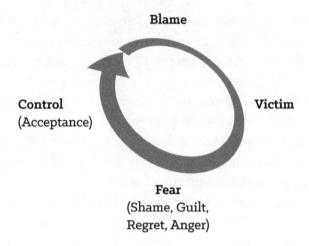

Blame

Control
(Acceptance)

Victim

Fear
(Shame, Guilt,
Regret, Anger)

Clearly, she's the problem, and she needs to change if your friendship is going to last. Step one, complete.

Next, you effortlessly move on to the second phase of the cycle: victimhood. You feel powerless to transform the situation and decide she is never going to change. You believe you have tried everything. Depending on how long this has been happening you might "forgive and forget" or "let it go and move on." Step three isn't far behind: fear. Maybe it is the fear of losing a good friend, missing out, or being seen as heartless. It sets in and becomes a constant companion, along with other victim-based emotions like shame, guilt, regret, and anger.

Your solution is found at step four: control and acceptance. What positive mantras or boundaries do you need to put in place to stop this perceived negativity from invading your space? After a few more exhausting cycles, you may tell yourself this friend is really not good for you. After all, you have a lot of stress going on in your life right now. You need high vibrations and positive vibes and can't afford to spend time with people who zap your energy. You accept that you can't change her, so maybe you'll decide to stop spending time with this friend altogether. Or you might conclude the two of you can still do lunch together, but you'll refuse to let her drag you into her drama. Or maybe you'll give it one last try and work on some breathing exercises to tame your emotions and find your happy place next time she tries to drag you down. One way or another, you'll seek some manner of control.

However, control is a temporary state and requires a lot of energy to maintain. It can't last forever. So it isn't long before your mental and physical boundaries are breached. The lid comes off and your bubbling anger bursts out. This is often an unconscious process. You unknowingly reenter the cycle as these instances become opportunities to get a blame fix.

At times during the Victim Cycle, it will look like your self-control is working. The relationship sees improvement. Perhaps you feel empowered and bathe in some much-needed respite. However, this relief is temporary because your blame addiction is still running unhindered below the surface. Eventually the tension will return. As much as you try to contain your annoyance or avoid someone, they will turn up somewhere and render your breathing exercises worthless. All to help you finally prove you were right—she is the problem and she needs to go!

Have you ever wondered why you are more sensitive and feel like you are being attacked at seemingly random times? Or why arguments occur when you are tired? The fact is, after a long day at work, a poor night's sleep, or a hard gym session, when your energy is low, you find it harder to maintain your self-control. You haven't got the energy to keep a lid on your honest emotions. So you're back to pointing the finger, and the cycle begins again. The only difference this time is that you are arguing over the smallest things like the dishwasher being packed in the wrong way. Whose fault is it that you weren't able to maintain control? Your spatially challenged partner? Your rubbish therapist? Your inconsiderate friend? Your ineffective breathing exercises? Yourself for not packing the dishwasher? More blame follows. Then more victimhood and fear. And another round of control. Avoidance follows until the final option is executed—separation. It is exhausting. This is why so many people feel like life resembles a relentless washing machine where we are waiting for the cycle to end so we can have a moment of peace before the next one begins.

Much of my work involves helping clients honestly heal from their blame addiction so they can exit the Victim Cycle. As they do, they no longer need the adrenaline and dopamine rush that comes with being in the washing machine. Profound transformations are then seen in all aspects of their lives. Relationships transform. Emotional reactions fundamentally change. Physical and mental pain and illness disappear. The impossible becomes possible. In time, as much as there can be uncomfortable moments, a deep sense of freedom and happiness becomes their new normal.

For example, one client started our sessions exasperated, expressing how he didn't know what to do with his youngest boy. His four-year-old son was a nightmare, he told me. The two of them regularly got into screaming matches and standoffs. It was the last straw when he found his phone in the toilet!

He was looking for help with some discipline tactics that would finally get the child under control.

My client had been going around the Victim Cycle for years with his son, and instead of feeding his blame addiction with more control-based tools and techniques, I did something very different. One of the ways of exiting the cycle is through igniting our curiosity. After a long time in the Victim Cycle, we learn to see the world as black and white. Curiosity to explore other possibilities opens us up to seeing in color again.

"What possible reason could there be for your son to drop your phone in the toilet?" I asked.

"Because he is a little shit!" the man blasted back at me. "Whatever I do to control his naughty behavior, nothing works. In fact, it seems to be getting worse."

My client was deep in his addiction and everything was in the firing line. At no point had he even considered the possibility that he was being a victim. He was blaming his son for being combative, hyper, and difficult. My client viewed himself as the poor helpless parent who was being run ragged by his disgraceful child. He had gotten to the point where he was looking for confirmation his son was the issue. Feeling like he had tried everything, he started looking for a child psychiatrist who could write a prescription, as he was convinced his boy had some type of ADHD, OCD, or some other label. My client was unknowingly looking for something else to blame, thinking that perhaps medication would once again give him back control of his life and kid. However, this strategy is just kicking the can down the road, where the can turns into a dumpster truck of pent-up issues looking for a place to dump it all on. Usually back on the parent.

To help clients start the process of exiting the Victim Cycle, I ask them to keep things simple. Because they are often in crisis mode, which comes with a lot of physical or emotional pain, everything seems very complicated. I said to my client, "Let's just look at the facts—your phone was in the toilet." So I asked my client to entertain the idea that he secretly wanted his phone to be out of action. Not necessarily at the bottom of his toilet but definitely out of action. He was struggling with the concept, so to help him I inquired about his life to get a bit more context.

He had told me how insanely busy he had been lately, so I asked, "Have you been spending more time on your phone?"

Yes, he admitted. The time he was spending on his laptop and phone had increased dramatically over the last eighteen months. He'd even been receiving comments from his wife and other children about being stressed, short-tempered, and distant.

As we spoke, it became obvious this man wasn't enjoying his life. He had an internal battle raging inside. He desperately wanted to spend more time with his family. But he was doing what he thought he was supposed to do: be the provider. He was playing his roles of "Husband," "Father," and "Provider" one-dimensionally. My client told me he fantasized about throwing his phone out the window many times and even acted this out as he told the story, something I knew he had done many times in front of his boy. So by throwing the phone down the toilet, his son did something that my client wanted to do himself but would never have dreamed of consciously doing.

When my client saw this symbolic act in a very different way, it had a huge impact. He admitted his growing frustration was bubbling over to all areas of his life. Friends and work colleagues were echoing the same message he was receiving from his family. Being in the Victim Cycle—blaming himself for not doing enough while blaming everyone else for not supporting him—had taken a toll. His body was hurting in ways it never had before, which he blamed on old age. Full of fear, shame, guilt, regret, and anger, he couldn't sleep. And after a while, even the extra espresso wasn't supporting him anymore.

As my client started to exit the Victim Cycle, he started to see how people had been helping in their own individual ways. It was not in ways he enjoyed, but nevertheless he could now see the love and intention behind their comments and behaviors. As for his four-year-old son, life's solutions were very simple—Daddy gets mad and shouts into his phone a lot and then doesn't play with me; I like playing with Daddy so I will get rid of the problem.

As my client went through the blame-recovery process, his relationship with his son changed. His need to control his son significantly lessened along with the fights. He was naturally and honestly empathetic instead of blaming, and listening instead of ignoring. The behavior problems and "acting out" changed in remarkable and effortless ways. The most astonishing change was that for the first time, his son asked to brush his teeth. My client was still visibly shocked as he recollected all the previous battles, morning and night, to get him to clean his teeth.

The simple truth is, it wasn't that his son didn't want to cooperate or even brush his teeth. He, like everyone else, didn't want to be ruled with an iron fist.

Reimagining Pain

When we have a small cut or a minor headache, it is easier to entertain the idea that the pain is a messenger. It motivates us to care for ourselves, cover up the wound, and maybe hydrate more. In the same way, if we are slightly irritated with someone it will be easier to understand they might be trying to help us. However, when we are swirling around in the Victim Cycle, it is easy to view any level of pain or irritation as bleak signs that the end of the world is nigh and everyone is against us.

Physical, emotional, and mental pain are messengers helping us take notice that something needs addressing. It is a logical process mimicking the butterfly effect, which theorizes that a flap of a butterfly's wing can later lead to a hurricane on the other side of the world. The imperceptible message alerts us to areas that are in need of attention, and the longer we ignore the signals the louder and more painful they become. Being dehydrated can go from dry lips to a headache to fainting, or kidney stones. Regardless of the intensity, hydrating can be the simple solution. Likewise, being irritated with your boss can soon escalate to a written warning before you are in each other's face looking for retribution. Again, addressing our blame addiction can be the simple solution. The sooner we do that, the less extreme our experiences become.

While we are in the Victim Cycle, we don't have access to this awareness. We just want the pain to STOP. Blaming whatever we think is the cause increases our fear, which prompts us to seek control. Before we know it, we are in another cycle of the washing machine wishing and hoping the pain will go away. If it doesn't, we accept that we are powerless to heal ourselves.

We defer responsibility and find something or someone to do the job for us. It is a natural response based on thousands of years being addicted to playing the Blame Game. It has led us to forget we are in fact profound self-healing organisms. Yes we need help, but, just like we are the ones that ultimately make ourselves angry or laugh, we are the ones that ultimately heal ourselves.

When we experience pain, we often find ourselves playing the second most prolific game: the waiting game. We wait and see before we take notice and look for help. We proudly claim, "It's nothing, I can barely feel it." This attitude might be very stoic and even respected, but it leads to more extreme symptoms. As much as we deep down know that our pain acts as a signal that will keep getting louder until we take notice, we've grown up in a culture that trains us to blame, ignore, push through, and silence our pain rather than learn its language and listen earlier.

As such, most of us have come to believe excessive pain, suffering, and hardship are inescapable aspects of human existence. We say things like, "Life's a bitch and then you die," "no pain, no gain," and "it's not always sunshine and rainbows." We wear pain and stress like a badge of honor. We even try to one-up each other's hardships, saying things like, "If you think that's bad, listen to this…" It seems pain and suffering simply come with living, and we just accept there's no escaping that fact. From broken hearts to financial instability, the message is clear: excessive pain is inevitable. In the immortal words of Rocky Balboa: "*You, me, or nobody is gonna hit as hard as life. But it ain't about how hard ya hit. It's about how hard you can get hit and keep moving forward.*"

Because we have accepted the *life is a battle* mantra, we also believe that the only way we learn is through pain and hardship. Some go so far as to say life would be boring if it was easy. This is only because they have never lived outside the Victim Cycle. They don't know any other version of reality. But just outside the circle is where we experience emotional states like honest curiosity, empathy, and joy, which all lead to optimal health, adventure, and wonderment. Life is very far from boring when you find meaning and experience a profound sense of freedom and effortlessness that result from the blame-recovery process.

The issue is that much of the rhetoric around happiness is steeped in stoic advice. So life becomes a fight as we attempt to forcefully change our perception and control and numb our pain. We search for the silver lining, pop Advil, get a cortisone injection, manage our expectations, live in the present moment, binge on ice cream, and watch endless streaming series—all in an effort to make ourselves feel better. When the effects wear off, we wonder what's wrong with us. Why are we still in pain, exhausted, unhappy, and unmotivated?

I lived this way until one synchronistic encounter changed my life forever.

Pain Is a Guide

Many moons ago, before I had the mindset I have today, I was caught firmly in London's rat race perfecting the *be the boss and master of your mind* mindset. I learnt to control my so-called demons and plough through my days. I thought I was performing well in my job and no one knew what was really going on behind my fake smile. Until I was unceremoniously called into my managers office at 8 p.m. and told I would need to find a new job. The train journey home to my girlfriend was a long one as I contemplated all the ways I could spin this into a positive. This was a profound life-changing moment, but it wasn't the synchronistic moment I am referring to.

I was surprised a few months later to find myself enrolled on a personal trainer course. Being thirty-one years old, this was very far from what I ever thought I would be doing at this age. The trepidation around my new career was palpable for my girlfriend, but she supported me all the way. Those fears were soon subdued a few weeks into my first position when a new client bought a block of sessions and gave me an envelope stuffed with two thousand pounds. It wasn't long before my smile became a little more honest and I was making more money than I did in my previous job.

This enabled me to travel the world learning all I could about strength and conditioning and nutrition. This initiated a passion. I had to know how the human body worked. I struggled with pain and didn't realize this would be the catalyst for what I would learn next. As a personal trainer, I looked healthy on the outside, but my body ached and I was experiencing emotional pain. I had no idea how my emotions were guiding me because I was too busy using exercise to keep them at bay. Based on my training I had an idea about what my physical pain was telling me, but I defaulted to the obvious reasons. I thought it was telling me to rest and lift lighter weights, so I did that. I thought my body needed different exercises, so that is what I did. None of it worked for long.

I sought out physios, osteopaths, and masseuses to help get rid of the pain. The pain always returned, so I decided to complete a sports massage course thinking that would not only alleviate the pain but give me another string to my bow to help my injured clients. Something strange happened. Instead of being disappointed that my pain remained, it ignited my curiosity to learn more about physical rehabilitation. I couldn't get enough. I read, listened, and watched all I could. Before I knew it, I had a ticket to Las Vegas, USA, to attend an innovative rehabilitation course. Normally you would have to be a qualified chiropractor to attend, but I messaged the organizer beforehand and detailed my learnings and skills and he agreed. I couldn't believe it. I was so excited.

A week before my flight I received an email telling me it was cancelled.

I was gutted! However, not for long. Since I was the only international participant, he understood the inconvenience this caused and offered me the opportunity to shadow him for three days at his clinic in Estonia. In the month that followed, I was like a child waiting to open their presents on Christmas morning. On the first day I got everything I asked Santa for and more. He had sent me manuals to study, and I was like the Cookie Monster from *Sesame Street* eagerly spending day and night consuming them. During the three days my passion and knowledge was obvious, and as such, he invited me to join the next training cohort being held in Miami, USA. Before I had returned home to the UK, I had a ticket to Florida booked.

A week before my flight I received an email telling me it was confirmed.

All my Christmases came at once. Little did I realize all these unexpected events would lead me to a life-changing synchronistic encounter. One morning with twenty minutes to spare before my class started, I was sitting on a beach, reading the course manual, when I heard, "Oh my, Mr. Murphy!" I looked up and there was an old university friend. I hadn't spoken to Helen in over fifteen years, and she happened to be taking part in a different course nearby. She invited me to attend a lecture that evening and catch up after. How could I say no after such a series of synchronistic events over the last few months to get me to that place at that exact time!

That night at the talk, a long-haired professor in a tie-dye button-down rambled on about life forces, energy work, and spiritual healing. I was furious Helen had tricked me into attending this complete waste-of-time presentation. I left midway through the lecture, making my disapproval known when I let the heavy auditorium door slam shut behind me.

I didn't reconnect with Helen that evening, but after a few curt text messages we agreed to meet for lunch the next day.

I went into our second encounter ready to shame my old friend for causing an incredibly disappointing night. While I was at it, I would prove my beliefs were right and hers were insane. Maybe I could even show her how stupid she was for paying a few thousand dollars to attend such a woo-woo seminar.

Helen joined me at the restaurant and I quickly attacked every point the crazy guy had made the night before. But she remained gracious. I couldn't rattle her at all. That one-hour lunch ended up stretching well into the evening. I heard about energy, frequency, vibration, epigenetics, synchronicity, quantum theory, soul contracts, past lives, the law of attraction, karma, forgiveness, acceptance, hope, positive mental attitudes, and more. Helen told me fantastical stories of shamans and healers helping people heal and transform—and through it all, something struck a chord. I was curious to know more.

Over the next five years I traveled around the world exploring these teachings for myself. I jumped in with two feet and experienced all I could in regards to healing and transformation. However, I was left wondering whether I was doing something wrong. I really went all in. I sold my house and car, ended a ten-year relationship with my girlfriend, gave away my possessions, and lived out of a backpack for those five years. But even though I went through periods of time where I felt fantastic, eventually the physical and emotional pain always came back with a vengeance. The issue was, I didn't realize until years later that the teachings, tools, and techniques I learnt were unknowingly feeding my unknown blame addiction.

It set me on a path to question everything I accepted as truth. It came with a lot of pain and struggle. But now, when I look back, the suffering was present because I was feeding my blame addiction at the same time as I was attempting to heal from it. I spent six years in a gym with the *no pain, no gain* attitude. Now I started to think about *no blame, no pain*. The issue was, I had no idea yet how blame had become so seamlessly interwoven into the very fabric of our language, society, and philosophical outlooks.

It soon became apparent that "healing" had become another word for control. People like myself were in fact just looking for the pain to stop so they could continue living in the same way as before. Not realizing, it was this way of living that brought about the pain in the first place.

Honest Healing

After over a decade of feedback from my life and my clients I can comfortably hypothesize that as we recover from our blame addiction, we have less emotional and physical pain as we experience fewer instances of feeling betrayed, treated unfairly, or held back. Life just seems to get more effortless. Like any new skill, it takes effort for it to become effortless. After thousands of years of dedicated practice, humans have become expert blamers and masterful victims. It is why feelings of fear, anger, shame, guilt, and regret have become so commonplace we think they are a natural part of being human, when in fact they are just the result of our blame addiction.

The honest healing process is about facilitating our innate ability to effortlessly self-heal. I am suggesting that recovering from our blame addiction is what allows our self-healing ability to become effortless.

It isn't about consciously forcing ourselves to STOP blaming. The forced approach doesn't yield long-term results for changing our habits or seeing our pain dissolve, so why would it work to help us recover from our blame addiction? It doesn't. This control-based approach results in ever more extreme situations because it just postpones what needs to be honestly healed.

Self-healing and rejuvenation occur when our need to blame naturally fades away as a by-product of us getting more deeply connected with our honest selves. That's why I classify this as a philosophy book rather than self-help. I am not selling a practice of manifestation, law of attraction, visualization, meditation, or affirmations to help you be more positive and eliminate blame from your life once and for all. I'm not offering empty platitudes or claims that you will instantly get everything you want by positive intention alone. There is no grand esoteric teaching or pseudo-empowerment rhetoric in this book that can be dismantled six months from now.

The approach I offer is very simple, but ironically it has taken me over a decade to put it into simple words. The honest self-healing journey will be different for everyone, which is why I won't say that it will be easy or that it will be hard. What I will say is that blame has been our constant and loyal companion for thousands of years. As we ween ourselves off our blame crutches, it might feel weird, confusing, unsettling, and frustrating at times. Even the feelings of profound freedom and liberation that replace it can feel strange and unfamiliar. But soon, some part of us remembers that it is our normal state. The way it was at some distant time in our past.

Exiting the Victim Cycle will require us to get uncomfortably honest. Not with others, but with ourselves. Honestly healing from this addiction is by no means for the faint of heart. But the journey is very much worth it. As your new awareness develops, you'll notice something a client of mine recently articulated very well. She said, "It's strange. I started to get that butterfly in the tummy feeling, like when you're first falling in love. But it didn't make sense because I was getting out of a relationship, not into a new one. Then I realized I was entering into a new relationship with myself." As your emotional, mental, and physical pain dissipates, a deep sense of self-worth and honest confidence fills the void. You relate to yourself, and then others, in a whole new way.

The Victim Cycle

When we talk about healing, there is often an assumption that something is broken. The premise is generally that somewhere along the line we got messed up and if we can fix it, we'll be all right again. When we honestly heal from our addiction to blame, however, we are not "fixing" anything. When I speak of healing, I'm using the word in its purest sense. We are always self-healing, and pain is not a sign we are damaged. It is simply a messenger letting us know that something needs addressing. We just have to get better at honestly listening to understand its language and experience how simple it can be to physically, emotionally, and mentally heal. As a sixty-year-old client told me after practicing this philosophy for a short while, "I don't wake up now and head for the medicine cabinet. I don't need painkillers anymore for the first time in eight years."

Healing from pain or any addiction has been made out to be an arduous task and often feels insurmountable. Our current approaches can make the journey of recovery feel like that of Sisyphus from Greek mythology. He was punished by Zeus and forced to roll an immense boulder up a hill, only to have it roll back down every time he neared the top. He was doomed to continue repeating this action for eternity. Healing only feels like this because we have been approaching it while unknowingly entrenched in the Victim Cycle, where control and acceptance have been our dominant tools.

We have been using much needed external and mental crutches to control and conquer our pain. But none of these have helped us heal the very foundation that is creating the pain in the first place—our blame addiction. Blame, like alcohol, sugar, and opioids, is not the enemy; it is our relationship with it that needs addressing. As blame becomes a less prominent feature in our lives, we experience less mental and physical pain. With less emotional pain, we have less need and desire for excessive alcohol, sugar, opioids, or whatever the addiction may be. Simply put, when we recover from our blame addiction, all other addictions effortlessly heal.

As control no longer becomes our go-to answer, we naturally become more self-honest and get closer to knowing who we honestly are. This is arguably the purpose of every human and why they are on Earth.

CHAPTER 3

The Control-and-Conquer Approach

While most people haven't considered the wide-ranging implications of playing the Blame Game, nearly everyone has an opinion on control. In general, it's thought of as something we should all strive for. Ironically, we may not like it when others control us, but most assert the benefits of controlling others or ourselves. We strive to control and conquer our feelings, our thoughts, and our bodies. We use self-control to curtail our spending, our eating, and our social media use. If we want to achieve greatness, the wisdom goes, we must first control-and-conquer ourselves.

The premise that self-control is admirable has lasted the test of time, from ancient Stoic philosophers to modern-day positive mindset gurus. If *control* is touted as the answer to our prayers, it seems logical that the lack of it is seen as the reason we are unhappy, unsuccessful, and unfulfilled. How can we question such wisdom?

> *"High self-esteem comes from feeling like you have control over events not that events have control over you."*
>
> —TONY ROBBINS

> *"It is better to conquer yourself than to win a thousand battles."*
>
> —BUDDHA

> *"For a man to conquer himself is the first and noblest of all victories."*
>
> —PLATO

> *"If you do not conquer self, you will be conquered by self."*
>
> —NAPOLEON HILL

> *"A disciplined mind leads to happiness, and an undisciplined mind leads to suffering."*
>
> —THE DALAI LAMA

The list of quotes is endless, but the notion is always the same: control and conquer yourself and you will be victorious in life. When such well-respected idols are in common agreement, it's wise to accept their wisdom and foolhardy to forgo their guidance, right?

But after going on my own search for meaning, spending years seeking a cure-all to my pain and lack of fulfilment, I finally questioned the unquestionable I'd previously accepted as truth. I wondered whether control is really all it's cracked up to be.

I learned about the incredible power of the human mind when I started practicing wing chun kung fu as a teenager and became fascinated with the Shaolin monks and their incredible superhuman feats of strength, endurance, and mobility. At the same time, I studied Bushido, the way of the samurai warrior. I heavily bought into self-control and the idea of becoming the master of my mind and body.

Honing my self-control gave me a sense of satisfaction and achievement to overcome one hurdle after another. I continued to collect personal evidence to prove mental toughness works and is the key to success. After all, we have to do things we don't want to in life, so we better get better at building resilience and mental calluses if we want to survive those tough times. My life seemed to mirror the ancient wisdom. At no point did it occur to me that those revered thinkers might have been unknowingly addicted to blame.

After seven years working in London's rat race and six years as a personal trainer, I was happy to have this ancient wisdom at my disposal. I wouldn't be here today without it. But after my synchronistic meeting with Helen in Miami, something changed in me. My mind opened. I didn't like it at the time because it took me way outside my comfort zone, but it gave me access to new information and awareness. My dormant curiosity came to life as I returned to London. I was thirty-six, and after selling my house and giving away most of my possessions, I found myself living on my friend's couch. I could have bought a new home. I could have gone back to the way things were and continued to build my personal training and physical rehabilitation business. But something in me wanted more. As my clients left, I didn't want to find new ones. You could say it was a slow burner followed by an epiphany, but I realized I needed healing! So I bought a backpack and a ticket to California in search of adventure, healing, and spiritual enlightenment.

In the years that followed, I sought the insights of boundary-pushing healers and philosophers. All their wisdom, tools, and techniques provided the intellectual stimulation I needed, and it felt incredibly satisfying. Yet, no matter how many changes I made and how good I initially felt as a result, I eventually found myself in the same painful and exhausted place.

Not deterred, I followed the latest neuroscience and reprogrammed, rewired, and reset my so-called negative thoughts and limiting beliefs that I was told were holding me back. While I could succeed in controlling and manipulating my mind for a time, the effects invariably waned. Then I would seek out a new healer or teacher and start the process anew.

With the help of my dogged determination, self-discipline, and self-control I kept telling myself, "This time it must be different! It has to get better. I've put in the work. I'm a good person. I deserve more!" Many times I felt I'd found the core issue as to why my life was so painful and taxing. I focused on the now to help me get rid of my so-called mental toxins such as greed, pride, hatred, obsession, and envy. However, as soon as I pulled myself up by the bootstraps, I would quickly find myself flat on my back, with less energy to stand up again.

I learned about Taoism, embraced *wu wei*, and went with the flow. I lived like a hermit, wandering the planet, spending time in isolation and meditation. I observed my thoughts and feelings. I stopped forcing action to get comfortable doing less. I practiced being patient. It felt amazing for a time. To go from busy to relaxing. But it wasn't long before I once again felt more frustrated. I learned so much from all that I was exposed to and had life-changing adventures as a result. I just didn't realize that these teachings and techniques had a foundation in blame and were based around control, which is why I remained swirling around in the Victim Cycle.

Many people think, like I did, that control, acceptance, and "letting go" is necessary to achieve success, happiness, and love. We convince ourselves if we could only control our perceived negative thoughts, emotions, and behaviors, then we would finally have the life we know we truly deserve. This mindset, which I refer to as the *control-and-conquer approach*, is extremely pervasive, but the side effects all around the world are showing us that it isn't a sustainable strategy for life.

The Way of the Control-and-Conquer Warrior

The idea that we should be able to control our minds to avoid painful emotions is prevalent in the media and among therapists and psychologists. We use words like "emotionally stable" and "emotionally intelligent" to describe cool, calm, and collected people who don't seem to experience many unpleasant feelings. We hold these people up as models of outstanding mental health.

Nearly all the self-help methodologies we have today are based on the control-and-conquer paradigm. Religion, spirituality, philosophical traditions, positive psychology, heart math, habit forming, the law of attraction, psychoanalysis, neuro-linguistic programming (NLP), affirmations, gratitude journaling, hypnosis, and cognitive behavioral therapy (CBT) are just a few examples. Each of these approaches and ideologies is predicated on one of the greatest myths we have ever been sold: the idea that our minds and brains (and souls) are malfunctioning and doing something wrong. As such, dividing our experiences into what we deem as rigidly positive and negative feels normal, while forcing change and consciously controlling our thoughts, emotions, and behaviors is seen as the solution.

Nowhere is this more prevalent then in the Stoic-inspired positive mental attitude movement, which promises the erasure of our so-called negative feelings if we just consistently compel ourselves to be positive. It promises we can "fake it 'til we make it," or reprogram ourselves through hypnotic daily practices such as mantras, affirmations, and gratitude journaling.

The popular *law of attraction* adopted this notion and suggests we must constantly think of what we want in order to attract it to ourselves. I was a devote, listening to Rhonda Byrne's book, *The Secret*, on repeat during my lunch breaks. However, I didn't realize the fear that was building under the surface each time I pressed play on the audiobook. I was afraid that I wouldn't apply the teachings correctly and the consequences would be dire. If I wasn't thinking, visualizing, or feeling the positive outcome of my desire enough, and thinking about possible *negative* outcomes, I'd attract negative events and toxic people into my life. It made sense based on thousands of years of exposure to this way of thinking. It has influenced so many of our modern-day success gurus. Recently I came across one who said: "When you are complaining, you are focusing on what is wrong in your life. Here is the universal law. What you focus on you move towards. You attract what you focus on. If you focus on all the shit, you become a shit magnet." It is hard not to accept this negative attracts negative, positive brings about positive line of thinking. They come with great sales pitches. But their solution to focus on the positive is wearing thin. Because this type of advice is steeped in blame, the pseudo-empowering feeling you get comes with a short shelf life.

We often accept the same advice around biohacking, weight loss, and entrepreneurialism. They all require a healthy dose of self-control as you are encouraged to strictly adhere to rules about how you should eat, sleep, and think. We are bestowed with wisdom that assures us we have to do things we don't like as we go through life. To make the journey more bearable, we are told to ignore and control our so-called self-sabotaging thoughts, desires, and habits and force ourselves to follow a certain morning or evening routine every day. Again, fear grows like mold in these environments because we worry that we won't be able to keep the new behaviors and habits going.

Control feels like a natural and logical thing to do, but we can't get away from the fact it is a short-term solution for any situation we are in. More importantly, for the purposes of helping explain how we can profoundly self-heal, it is silencing our honest desires, thoughts, and feelings. It keeps us in a state of dishonesty, mostly with ourselves. Because we haven't been listening to them all our life, they become amplified to get our attention. Our self-honesty has been yelling, waiting for us to listen. But we can't hear it while we are being a control-and-conquer warrior.

Control Isn't the Enemy

At first it feels great to know we can always use control and push through our discomfort and check the next item off our to-do list. Snoozing when you have a work assignment due in the morning? Change your inner state, listen to a motivational podcast, and polish off that report with flying colors. Stuck on the couch when you promised yourself you'd start working out? Gaze into the mirror, grab a handful of belly fat, and get your lazy ass to the gym to sculpt those abs. All these tactics work, but are they sustainable?

Just as blame isn't the enemy, neither is control. We only have to look at people like Arnold Schwarzenegger to see how the control-and-conquer approach can help us achieve our goals. Arnold became Mr. Olympia multiple times by working out twice a day for six days a week and consuming enough raw eggs and chicken breasts to feed a family of four to gain muscle mass. Thanks to positive affirmations and a positive mental attitude, he was able to push through the pain and achieve his goals. Similarly, Joe Simpson became famous after recounting his epic story of how he stayed alive after a horrific incident while climbing Siula Grande in the Peruvian Andes in the book *Touching the Void*. Digging deep to control our desire to give up can help us reach seemingly impossible goals. We have amazing untapped reserves to achieve extraordinary feats.

It is unquestionable that self-control showcases what humans can do. But what are the side effects? Is it healthy to eat and train in these extreme ways? Just because you lived through an extreme situation, can you do it again and again? Is it a sustainable strategy for life? And could this reserve of energy be directed somewhere else for even greater potential?

Many entrepreneurial influencers like Gary Vaynerchuk, Kylie Jenner, and Grant Cardone have utilized a control-and-conquer approach to hustle and grow their business empires. The message they send to the rest of us is that we should push through the pain too. We only have ourselves to blame if we don't man up, put our warrior faces on, and get more positive. We should learn better life hacks and try harder to stick to our rigid habits.

This approach to life feeds our addiction to blame by assuming we have the power to choose how we feel at any given moment. If we are feeling pain or discomfort, it is our own fault for not getting rid of those feelings. We should just snap out of it and let it go.

We are told seemingly empowering nuggets of wisdom like, "There are things you can control and things you can't, so focus on the ones you can." We latch onto these ideas. They feed the whole notion that control is the answer, not realizing the place we focus control will become the most stressful part of our life. Just like my client who controlled his kid and found his phone in the toilet along with his home life—he thought he couldn't control his workflow and boss, so he accepted that and redirected it to his family.

It can also feel good to be told, "You can't always control what happens to you, but you can always control your response." Again, it seems empowering. But what is this actually teaching us?

How To Get Better at Blaming

Based on what we went through in chapter one, this control-and-conquer approach is ingraining the blame-based idea that others are responsible for why we feel the way we do. When in fact, our feelings have nothing to do with what others do or say. It is our sense of victimhood that influences how we perceive and interpret what others do or say. So the fact you found someone annoying or feel hurt by something they said isn't a representation of what actually occurred. You blamed them, felt like a victim, lost "control," and then your honest feelings of disappointment and anger revealed themselves. You unconsciously used the other person as a valve to *let off steam*.

Even if you still think others are responsible for your emotional state, is it true that you can *always* control your response? You might be able to for long periods of time if you have developed Navy SEAL–level self-control. But even the Navy SEAL can burn out and be labeled with PTSD at some point, because their mental stability was based on the illusion of control.

It is worth reiterating—the whole control-and-conquer approach to life is predicated not only on the myth that things are going wrong, but also on the premise we make conscious decisions. In fact, as will become more evident as you make your way through this philosophy, our decisions originate from whatever is in our foundation and our conscious mind just executes them. If your foundation is full of blame addiction, victimhood, fear, and anger, then your perception and experience of the world will reflect this. What you eat, watch, and partake in is a reflection of what is in your foundation, not a conscious decision.

As you start to recover from your blame addiction, your foundation becomes full of love, curiosity, and empathy. As a result, your perceptions and decisions effortlessly change. You want to eat differently. You want to move and be more creative. You start to discover who you honestly are—along with dreams and passions you didn't realize you had. It results in us feeling energized rather than exhausted.

When our ability to control something runs its course, we resort to the last form of control we have available to us: *acceptance*. Some happiness gurus proclaim the answer is *radical acceptance*, not realizing this is just another phrase for *radical control*. And without realizing it, acceptance acts like Kryptonite to superman—it renders us powerless. If I want to get this across to a client, I say something I know they won't like to accept. For example, if I am talking with a high-powered female executive who is working in the tech industry, I can guess the journey she has had. The technology industry has been a male-dominated field for a long time, and so she would have had to push through many "glass ceilings" to achieve her success. I will look her in the eyes and say something like, "Just *accept* that you will never be as good and successful as a man."

More often than not, she will react like a cobra feeling threatened. Every cell of her body wants to break out of the mental prison I just put her in. The concept of *acceptance* is only used and promoted by victims. People who have given up on all other possibilities. I know every one of the Paralympians didn't accept their diagnosis from a doctor that they will never walk, run, swim, throw, jump, or play their sport again. Acceptance is very powerful, but not in the way it has been sold. It feeds our blame addiction and keeps us confined to the life of a victim.

It is a concept that keeps us spinning once again in the Victim Cycle. To stop the pain, we become seduced by more blame-fueled advice. It comes in many forms: "You can choose to be a victim or you can choose to take control." "STOP blaming others. Be responsible for your actions, learn from your mistakes, and move on." "Write a different narrative to your victim mentality." "Flip the script to a more positive one."

Because these types of advice have the word blame and victim in them, it is thought I am saying the same thing. I get sent quotes and videos often saying, "This person is saying the same as you." However, nothing could be further from the truth. I understand why it happens because I said I am offering something different, and this can be a challenging thought considering all the past wisdom we have available to us at our fingertips. As I mentioned in chapter 1, I am offering an alternative, not the truth. I have just recognized that the sentiment emanating from this type of advice is firmly rooted in the control-and-conquer mindset, which ultimately keeps us in the Victim Cycle.

When we stumble in our ability to control ourselves or our environment, we search around for something to blame and seek to get back in control. This path is paved with pain and disappointment because we are seeking an illusion. Control is a mirage and it keeps us lost in the desert. We keep thinking we are almost there, but the oasis never arrives. At some point we accept our fate, *it is what it is*, and then seek out more powerful sedatives.

Imagine a man stuck in this cycle. He is stuck in traffic. The man is upset, but he controls his anger and reprimands himself for not leaving home sooner. How silly of him to forget to plan for potential delays! He makes it to his recreational soccer game in an agitated state, only to collide with another player and hurt his knee. He immediately blames himself for being careless while internally grumbling at the other player for not being more mindful. But he controls his feelings, and like a proper man he continues to play on. By the end of the game, he is in excruciating pain and heads to the hospital, where he finds out he will need surgery. Behind his brave face, his honest feelings of blame, victimhood, fear, and anger bubble up, which sends his need for control into overdrive.

Because he has used a lot of energy to hide his honest emotional state, he is unable to control his frustration and anger any longer. That evening he snaps at his wife. She assumes her husband's short temper must be a result of his pain, so she matches his bravado by smiling and keeping quiet. She decides to "walk on eggshells" to minimize the chances of upsetting him even further.

This *not wanting to make things worse* strategy looks supportive but is actually part of the Blame Game. His passive-aggressive comments turn into yelling. Soon a full-blown argument has started, and it continues for days. Each blames the other. Both look to assert their victimhood in their own way. Because the children are being affected, they decide to bury the hatchet and make up. The valves were opened, the pressure was released, and now all is back to normal. But what is normal? How long will they control themselves this time before the next blame eruption?

The challenge is that we're often unaware that blame and victimhood are actually at the root of our desire to control things. We see control as a helpful and admirable quality. We envy people who seem to have everything under control in their lives. And we all reinforce these ideas, pulling each other deeper into the blame addiction without even realizing it.

In a world saturated with blame, the control-and-conquer approach is the only solution we have to get what we want.

Because humans are very creative, resilient, and resourceful beings, we constantly come up with new and improved ways to elicit more control. But control is temporary. And it is exhausting.

Built on a Foundation of Blame

Keeping everything in our lives under control sounds great in theory, but it requires a lot of effort to maintain. Eventually we run out of energy and realize we were never really in control in the first place. We were just keeping a lid on things, postponing the inevitable conflict and drama that comes with whirling around in the Victim Cycle.

One client in particular was experiencing the temporary nature of control very acutely. This man came to me after attending various seminars taught by some of the top self-help gurus on the planet. After each new workshop, he was able to better accept what he couldn't control and focus on what he thought he should control—his emotions. For a while, he experienced a period of what he described as "radical responsibility" and "radiant positivity." However, these periods had been getting shorter and were feeling harder to attain.

A few months prior, he attended a motivational workshop that taught him a handful of new ways to reframe his past and reprogram his thoughts so he could be more accountable and get more positive. The speaker played loud music and encouraged the audience to adopt a powerful stance, scream, dance, high-five, smile, and jump around. When everyone was thoroughly pumped up, the speaker told his listeners they could access this level of positivity at any time.

"We all just completely changed our inner state in sixty seconds," my client told me, "and the quicker we nip our negative headspace in the bud, we can have this feeling anytime we want. We never have to settle for feeling low, lazy, sad, angry, stressed, or frustrated. We are in control of our emotions; they aren't in control of us."

"That's a pretty common approach in the self-help world," I said. "And how's that working out for you?"

"Amazing," he forced out.

"Really?" I questioned. His energy, body language, and tone were reflecting back a very different story.

"Well," he shrugged, "if I am going to be honest, it is getting harder to force myself into that positive state. I don't think I'm doing it right. I have gotten caught up in work recently, but maybe I just need to practice the techniques more. I don't know…"

He was displaying groupthink and reciting what he had been told many times, telling himself that his emotions were wrong and it was his own fault he couldn't stop feeling them. Years of hearing about the importance of developing the *right* kind of attitude had fed the self-blame part of his addiction. The speaker swore these techniques worked for some of the world's richest people, so if they weren't working for my client, then his failures must be his own fault. He had been blamed that he didn't want to or wasn't ready to change. His fear and disappointment were palpable even though he thought he was doing a good job of hiding it.

The control-and-conquer approach is unknowingly built on a foundation of blame. Therefore, it doesn't lead to honest healing and long-term happiness. It is the reason why some of the world's richest people are depressed and on medication.

When we read about controlling our emotions, it sounds right. *Yes! That seems like exactly what I need!* It resonates with us. But why? Because it is feeding our addiction without us knowing it. Like any addiction, the message that we are not in a sustainable relationship will get louder and louder. Control is a temporary life strategy. Maintaining it requires an increasing amount of energy. Eventually, we can't sustain it any longer and our blame addiction bursts through, often in surprising and scary ways.

Many people have become rich and famous from teaching different ways to develop self-control and be positive to win the day, week, month, or year. But in the end, the control-and-conquer approach leaves us physically, mentally, and emotionally exhausted. Including the teachers and promoters of these strategies.

Pushing Through the Pain

The control-and-conquer approach seems empowering. It offers a simple solution, and we feel productive while in this space. We can achieve anything we want, the wisdom goes; we just need to identify our negative thought patterns and write ourselves some new, more positive ones to replace them. It gives us a clear and straightforward path to a better life. It allows us to take quick action and see some immediate results.

But at their core, these strategies are about repressing honest thoughts and forcing ourselves to think in a different (dishonest) way. As soon as you engage with this approach, you are blaming that thought or belief for being bad or negative.

So you might be able to sweep it under the rug, but it is still there regardless of what you do. No amount of rewiring, reprogramming, or resetting will erase it regardless of what the latest neuroscience hypnotic technique will tell you. The reality is that you now have two opposing thoughts running on top of each other. And when you run out of energy to keep the new one going, the old honest one leaps out from under the rug.

Making yourself chant positive affirmations can pump you up to nail your presentation. Working around the clock when your body desperately wants to sleep can lead to getting the big promotion. Starving yourself when you'd rather be gorging on fried chicken and waffles can help you lose weight and look slim in your wedding dress or movie role. But what happens after the event? Many newlyweds and actors laugh about their inability to maintain the level of self-control needed to keep the body they spent so much time sculpting.

Ignoring the pain and trying to push through the exhaustion leads to burnout. Many artists and business icons write books and give speeches on this very topic. Even if you can work late into the night and gain success at work, your relationships or hobbies might be affected. Other areas of your life will reflect your honesty and exhaustion. It is why so many people manage to be positive at work and bring about huge results, but they find themselves arguing more with their families. Those honest thoughts and feelings, the ones constantly pushing up against the rug, have to come out some time. Otherwise, the internal pressure and stress start to impact our mental and physical health. And before long, the same honesty and exhaustion will start to seep through at work. This isn't a fault in the design. It is to show us where we are blaming so we can start the recovery process and experience what true freedom feels like.

A recent client was in complete denial that he liked feeling in control. He had dedicated over two decades to self-development, reaching high levels of neuro-linguistic programming and many other modalities. He managed to control his emotions to such a level that he believed his own story about how laid back he was, and he prided himself on going with the flow. It was a eureka moment, albeit an uncomfortable one, when he realized his stress and exhaustion stemmed from the tight grip with which he ruled his behavior and familial relationships.

It felt so natural for him to control himself and others, he was oblivious to how much blame and victimhood he was swimming in. Any emotion he saw as negative and harmful to his goals was quickly dealt with and shut behind a door. They were out of sight, but not quite as out of mind as he thought. They were still part of him and affecting his health, business, and happiness. He told me his six-year-old son acted like a mischievous teenager and behaved terribly, doing the opposite of everything he asked and needing help with even the simplest of tasks, even though he had already mastered them.

Many parents create systems of rewards and punishments to incentivize their children to behave in certain ways and not in others. Whereas prison officials are happy to acknowledge their adherence to a control-and fear-based regime, parents are often in denial that they might be wardens overseeing a similar environment. They deny this even though solitary confinement is a common punishment—their children are banished to the bedroom or naughty step for misbehaving while extra time to play outside or watch TV is often a reward.

It was a year-long journey to help my client gain a different relationship with control. But watching his environment respond with each step motivated him to continue. Following one of our sessions, he was flabbergasted when his chronic back pain disappeared and didn't return. He thought people and situations in his life had always been trying to "hold him *back*" from his dreams. He was on a mission to prove them wrong. Without realizing it, his blame was stored in his back. It is the same as someone complaining that their brother is "a pain in the neck" while they vigorously rub their chronic neck tension. The messages are there; we just have to learn how to listen in a different way. And sometimes a simple change in our awareness and language is all that is needed to start the self-healing process.

Many of my clients come to me for help at a time in their life where they are frustrated and feel exhausted mentally, physically, and emotionally. They have read many stories about control leading to incredible survival and success stories. But they don't understand why they consistently feel so unhappy, unmotivated, and exhausted after following the same advice. They wonder why they can't just "be positive" like the books say. They have been told happiness is a choice and are frustrated as to why it's so difficult to make that choice every day. It used to work, but now it doesn't anymore.

As I mentioned before, this is because life isn't about making a conscious decision to be motivated, happy, or calm. If it was, there would be no issues or addictions in the world. We would simply do all the right things all the time. Our conscious mind doesn't create our decisions, it actions them. As we exit the Victim Cycle, our thought process and decisions naturally change because the elements that make up our foundation change. We then become very aware that control as the solution is energy draining, when life is designed to be energy generating.

The control-and-conquer approach requires a lot of energy at the start and even more effort to maintain. It is not an efficient strategy, but it is the only one we know. We think self-control is helping us achieve some type of freedom and that losing control is our problem. We can become so entrenched in this ideology we miss the fact that successful people like Arnold Schwarzenegger have found what they honestly want to do. They have found passion and meaning unique to them. This is what sustains them—not control, even if they think it is the key to success. Many who try to replicate his success don't reach the same level because they are forcing themselves to chase money or some other dishonest goal. One that doesn't match their genuine desire. So disappointment and burnout are the all-too-common side effects.

Forcing yourself to do something you honestly don't want to do will inevitably lead to burn out.

Burning Out

The constant pursuit of control is like holding a bar of soap in the shower: the tighter you grip, the more it slips out of your hand.

Running out of energy to keep everything under control is so common we actually have a phrase for it: "falling off the wagon." This is what we say has happened to the Mormon who defects from a lifestyle of strict control and becomes a chain-smoker addicted to his Tinder account. In the same way, an addict is accused of "relapsing" when they fall prey to temptation.

Many times I have been asked, "So if control-and-conquer is so bad, what am I supposed to do? Just go with the flow and hope for the best? Let my dog run around the house? Let my employees come into work whenever they want? Tell everyone how depressed I feel today?" This is the blame addiction kicking in. Jumping to the extreme end of the spectrum is a symptom of the Victim Cycle. It creates black-and-white thinking. More options exist, but we won't have access to them while we are in a state of victimhood and control.

If we look at many tech moguls, celebrities, and motivational entrepreneurs, we can see evidence of control-and-conquer at work. And these people are dripping with culturally verified success. Again, Grant Cardone has built a real estate business worth hundreds of millions. Kylie Jenner sits atop a massive makeup empire. Gary Vaynerchuk has used the control-and-conquer approach to build his massive social media following. GaryVee, as he is known on Twitter, has encouraged people to post on all social media outlets multiple times per day. It doesn't matter if you don't feel like posting today. According to his ethos, you need to work around the clock and get exposed to as many people as possible.

Similarly, if you're looking to become an Olympic athlete like Michael Phelps or Simone Biles, based on the control model, you are going to have to push through massive amounts of pain to get there. You'll need to stick to your strict diet and aggressive training plan, rain or shine. You won't always feel like following the schedule from your coach, but you must stick to it if you want to win.

Control isn't the enemy; it obviously has merit. But because it is a constant in our lives whether we know it or not, we haven't explored what human potential is available without it. We have examples of what is possible when we study people who have been diagnosed with "acquired savant syndrome." These people wake from trauma-induced comas to find themselves possessing incredible dormant skills they never knew they had. They might be anomalies, but like Siamese twins or the people featured in the *Stan Lee's Superhumans* TV show, they definitely deserve our curiosity.

What we do know is that when we adopt a control-and-conquer approach, success can arrive as our physical and mental health is impacted. It takes an incredible amount of effort to sustain fake happiness and keep our painful emotions at bay. It can often appear that running a business, raising a family, and staying in good physical shape are all stressful pursuits. But maybe it's really the maintenance of a control-and-conquer approach that is creating much of the excess stress that leads to exhaustion and illness. Maybe it is the underlying blame addiction and the idea that we need to force positivity and rigid habits that is wearing us down.

Nearly all wildly successful people eventually slow down and take a break at some point in their lives. GaryVee has taken time off from social media more than once. Simone Biles and Michael Phelps, like many athletes, admit to mental health issues.

No matter how the latest advice on happiness is packaged, the underlying message is always that we must corral our emotions, control our mind, and force a smile onto our faces whenever we can. But as I followed the leading self-help gurus closely over the past few decades, I noticed that they rarely adhere to this same mentality for long. Eventually they burn out from the effort of trying to stay outwardly happy and they change their tune. When they are first on the scene, they rave about how important it is to work around the clock to be successful. We must build up our reserves of willpower so we can avoid bad temptations and set good habits, they say. And then a few years down the line, they take a break from the heavy self-promotion and come back with a story about the importance of self-care, spending time with loved ones, and working smart rather than hard.

They often blame their breakdown on the fact they are "just human" or "still on the journey and still learning." But actually, they have just been playing the Blame Game without knowing it. And they needed a pause in the cycle to rejuvenate before they reentered the next cycle. They had become exhausted by their own advice.

There are schools of thought that recognize control isn't the answer and prefer to "go with the flow" instead. It sounds progressive and most definitely helps reduce surface-level stress. However, if we were on a river just going with the flow, where could we end up? It might be exhilarating to go through some rapids, but what if you are heading for a waterfall? Similarly, it might feel peaceful to hang out in the reeds, but at what point do you start feeling lost or stuck?

Because an alternative hasn't been offered, we cling firmly to the control-and-conquer approach, even when our mind, body, and relationships indicate a new approach is needed. We continue to patch up the gaps in our everything-is-fine, I-don't-care-what-people-think mindset with control-based habits, tools, and techniques. It is worth pondering what it would look like if we didn't become reliant on control. At first it might feel like a daunting prospect. But even if it feels uncomfortable, or we think mayhem would ensue, maybe there are other possibilities to explore.

CHAPTER 4

The Roots of Our Addiction

My sister was in time-out because our mother had noticed the bright red bite marks on my arm. But my sister hadn't bitten me. For several weeks, I had been biting *myself* whenever my older sister teased me. I learned that if I cried and pointed the finger, my mother would rush in to save the day. At five years old, I had already seen blame working in our family dynamics and so I cooked up a masterful plot to use it to my advantage. I suddenly had the power to make her stop picking on me, and it felt good.

The success didn't last for long, of course. My mother soon caught on to what I was doing, and I received my comeuppance. But by then, I'd learned that blame and victimhood are tools we can all use for getting what we want.

Our inherited blame addiction gets enforced early in life. And we learn that *it works*. Sure, it doesn't work for long, but that doesn't stop us from trying. And when it stops working, we don't even notice because we are already blaming our problems on the next thing.

When we are young, everyone teaches us to blame. Parents, teachers, older siblings, TV characters, and celebrities all preach the victimhood gospel. Imagine a small child bumping into a table and crying. Often, an adult will stand up, slap the table, and say, "Bad table!" The kid thinks this is silly, and it may even distract them from the pain. If it doesn't work, we encourage them to hit the table for themselves and repeat, "Bad table!" I remember doing this very thing with my nieces when they were children, and they would immediately stop crying, giggle, and continue with their play.

After successfully making my nieces feel better, I was too busy patting myself on the back for being a great uncle to notice I was actually giving the girls a master class in blame. Soon they would become blame prodigies and learn to cast themselves in the victim role effortlessly without my help. And what's more, without realizing it, by getting them to hit the table, I had taught them that when they feel emotionally or physically hurt, they should lash out.

As we transition to adulthood, our blaming outbursts feel righteous. They become second nature. We label others as "toxic" or "narcissistic" without realizing we are casting blame, deep in the throes of an addiction. Like any skill, the more we diligently practice this, the better we get. We are learning to be expert blamers from a young age. By the time we mature, our morals, values, and language are so infused with blame that we don't even notice it.

It's not only our parents, guardians, mentors, and peers who help us get our blame fix; we also learn to blame ourselves. We beat ourselves up for not being able to play catch like our brother. We feel bad for hurting Dad's back when he picked us up. We scold ourselves for being stupid because we failed another math test. We think if we were prettier or had longer hair, we would have a boyfriend. Self-blame is prolific and eventually shows itself as shame and guilt, which chips away at our self-worth and later impacts our physical and mental health.

Just as a fish doesn't know it is swimming in water, we don't realize we are constantly drenched in blame. It is the undercurrent that feeds our motivations and decisions. This turns into a self-perpetuating cycle. Popping painkillers to take away menstrual cramps so we can power through the day seems innocent enough. The medicine temporarily reduces the pain and even tempers our growing irritation. But we don't realize that in going down this path we've also subscribed to the subtle message of blaming our body and hormones for doing something wrong and causing our subpar ability to focus. So now we've become a victim of our monthly cycle. Even something as natural as the menstrual cycle is used to get our blame fix.

I remember getting some very strange looks from a group of women while I explained that the menstrual cycle is not meant to be painful. I mentioned that women commonly use it as an excuse to do what they honestly want to do. For instance, they might take some time out from a busy household, stay in for the evening to pamper themselves, or even use it to get some time off work. As I started to mention that both men and women have been taught to resort to blame and victimhood at this time of the month, one woman showed her outrage.

"How dare you," she exclaimed. "I *have* to take painkillers every month. Sometimes I need five or six just so I can function!"

The others nodded and the general consensus was, *How dare this man talk about what he doesn't have to endure every month.*

I explained that most of my clients are women. And the large majority of them report changes in their monthly cycle as a by-product of exiting the Victim Cycle. They tell me they've experienced a profound shift, whether this means they now feel zero pain, are regular, or have a greater feeling of lightness. It sounds unbelievable, but when we become aware how tense and contracted we are in the Victim Cycle, it makes sense that we expand and relax as we break free.

It is fair to say there is a lot of stigma, comedy, and pain associated with this time of the month. In some traditions a woman is seen as "unclean" or "dirty" during this time and is banned from entering religious places or gatherings. These and other blame-based ideas and traditions feed our sense of victimhood and increase the level of pain and discomfort.

I am not blaming parents, doctors, or religious traditions. And I am not blaming blame. We have been cultivating a global society of expert blamers and masterful victims and we have inherited this from our long-ago ancestors. It has been going on for such a long time, humans are now acting as one superorganism—a super victim. I am not blaming our ancestors either. To blame anyone or anything for our addiction would be perpetuating the Victim Cycle.

I am not even saying that the Victim Cycle should be blamed. Whirling around in this loop is not a sign you have somehow "failed." Having an addiction is also not a badge that reads "I could have tried harder." Addictions are simply an incessant message to become aware that we have been living with a victim mindset, even if we have controlled ourselves enough to think we are not. Our relationships with each other, ourselves, and nature would be very different if we had a different relationship with blame.

I would like to live in a world where sexual, physical, and psychological abuse of any kind are no longer part of our reality. These are all extreme symptoms of our blame addiction and the feelings of victimhood, fear, shame, and guilt that follow. I know this version of reality is possible because I see evidence everyday of what happens when we exit the Victim Cycle. To recover from our blame addiction and achieve a new superorganism, we must become more aware of where blame is hiding in our everyday vocabulary, thoughts, platitudes, idioms, concepts, and nuggets of advice.

The Tradition of Blame

We have been blaming, casting ourselves as victims, seeking control, and perpetuating the Victim Cycle since the dawn of recorded history. We've kept the cycle going because victimhood comes with short-term benefits. A big insurance payout can come from a burned-down house or factory. Breaking a vase will come with less repercussions if you hurt yourself at the same time. Being "clumsy" and tripping can defuse an awkward situation.

Blame is a paradox. On one hand it ultimately leads to physical, emotional, and mental pain. On the other hand, it can be painfully funny to watch a comedy show where everything is seemingly going wrong and people are getting hurt. Isn't this paradox the reality of every other addiction? Alcohol can provide the fuel for connection, laughter, and relaxation. But at what point does the fun turn into pain?

This confusion over blame's role is especially troubling for kids who do not yet possess the discernment or critical thinking capabilities to understand the nuances. When is it funny to blame, and when is it contributing to conflict? Why is it okay for a Marvel superhero to blame the villain and smash them into oblivion in a comical way but it's not okay for a child to lash out at Dad for turning off the TV?

To make blame even more baffling, there are cultural differences at play. People in one country consider it rude not to remove your shoes when entering a building. But citizens of a nearby country think it's strange to walk around shoeless. Our parameters for blame are always in flux. This is confusing even for adults. We often find ourselves playing the Blame Game even though we know it isn't the ultimate answer to life's issues. Because there hasn't been an alternative, we think of blame as essential for solving problems. However, it eventually leads to more extreme versions of the same problem.

Because blame is paradoxical, our goal is to change our relationship with blame rather than defeat it. Take a common scenario like waking up in the morning with a painful neck. Our first reaction might be to blame the pillow. Case solved. So what is the solution? Easy—jump online and shop for the latest innovation in pillow design. But what if we can't afford a new futuristic pillow? Now our only option is to suck it up and hope for the best. The end result of blame is a closed mind. It shuts down our curiosity and creativity, leaving us with only two viable choices. We can either replace the thing we see as causing our problem, or we can put up with the discomfort.

This solution cycle isn't really any different to when we blame our boss, friend, or partner for being the reason we are unhappy. Depending on how deep we are in the Victim Cycle, we can either get a new job or partner, or continue to put up with them and practice self-control. When we blame something for causing our unhappiness or pain, we narrow our focus down to these basic options, none of which are sustainable as they ultimately lead to denial, avoidance, and separation.

This victim mindset leads us to direct our focus away from what really matters—us and our blame addiction. It is why our medical system is constantly chasing symptoms. By blaming parts of our body for doing things they supposedly aren't meant to be doing, we enter the blame-based solution cycle. Either keep putting up with the discomfort, numb the pain, or become laser focused on getting rid of the perceived reason for the pain. As a young boy I used to get a lot of throat infections. The go-to solution at the time was to blame the tonsils and surgically remove them. However, this is like cutting out a partner from your life because you blame them for being the reason you are miserable. You might enjoy the relief, but how long is it before the same issues arise again? My throat infections might have subsided, but the reason for them showed up in different places in my body. This surgical procedure is less common now because the doctors have more information, awareness, and wisdom at their disposal. As great as it is they now realize the tonsils are not the problem, their "wisdom" still has a foundation in blame. So they are still looking for the next organ to remove or replace rather than helping the patient heal themselves.

The bigger-picture issue is not our uncomfortable pillow, inconsiderate partner, overbearing parent, or bullying boss. These are merely symptoms of something deeper. In retrospect, I can see how my inflamed tonsils were an indication of my raging anger, which I repressed most of the time using immense self-control. I wanted to scream my frustrations (blame) to the world, but I didn't. Because I no longer had tonsils to reflect my blame and anger, I "suffered" from painful mouth ulcers to give me another opportunity to heal. But of course, I had no idea how to do that so I continued to blame, get more angry, and get more ill.

Maybe our neck is stiff in the morning to bring attention to the argument we had the night before. Rather than rush to buy a new pillow, we might take a moment to realize our old one didn't go "bad" overnight. It might be the fact we are stressed after an evening blaming our brother for why we are unhappy. Similarly, we might want to look at other possibilities before we curse out our parent, break up with our partner, or hand in our resignation to our "bullying" boss. There might be some painful truths hidden in their comments. As we will discuss in much more detail later, the "labels" in our life very much impact what we see and hear. What seemed like insults, criticisms, or discouragement might be considered constructive feedback coming from someone else. When our "mum" or "boss" say something, it can sound completely different from when our "friend" or "coach" say exactly the same thing.

Many of my clients complain about back pain. Sometimes they blame it on sitting too much. Other times they attribute it to standing all day. Or they might have other targets for their blame-based analysis, like they don't stretch enough, haven't done yoga in a while, or "tweaked something" at the gym. These cause-and-effect stories make logical sense, but only because our reasoning is steeped in blame, victimhood, and fear. It won't feel like this to my clients as they assure me their pain is because of whatever they blamed. They will tell me, "After sitting all day, when I stretch or do yoga the pain goes." Or, "My back went out when I deadlifted more than I normally do." It is hard to argue with such a simple two plus two equals four equation.

Ultimately, as soon as we point the finger, our creativity and curiosity shut down, along with all other doors of possibility, leaving just two open. Suck it up and power through the day or gym session, or stop sitting and exercising altogether. Neither of which is a healthy or sustainable option.

But what if they only noticed the pain on stressful days? What if there were days they sat for longer and felt fine? What if they deadlifted a larger amount of weight to impress a friend or their trainer? Maybe it was what they were thinking while sitting or lifting that created tension in their body. And it is this that impacted their biomechanics rather than the actual activity being the issue…maybe?

When we are in the blame cause-and-effect mindset, at some point our victim response demands instant gratification: "Just take away the pain so I can get on with what I need to do." This mentality is rampant because the more entrenched we get in the Victim Cycle, the more adverse we become to emotional and physical pain. However, as will become evident later in the book, it is from respecting and listening to our pain that honest healing is achieved and freedom experienced.

Part of the reason our blame- and victim-based reasoning makes logical sense is because we have accepted the mainstream narrative that humans are innately made "for survival." Surviving, by definition, means we are just getting by while we find ways to cope with the daily slog of a tough existence. One article I came across was entitled, "Your brain's biological negative tendencies along with misguided belief systems create a recipe for tricking you out of success and into the safety of mediocracy." It is a mouthful that might resonate, but why? Because it is infused with blame. It is blaming your brain for holding you back from reaching your goals.

This would be a shitty design if the very thing you take everywhere with you was doing all it could to trick you into mediocracy. Or to simply focus on perceived negative and wrong outcomes. It feels like we are being tricked and held back, because it is an easy blame-based conclusion. So it is an easy way to get our blame fix.

Humans are innately collaborative, creative, and curious and designed to move regularly in a myriad of ways, all of which are the characteristics of species that want to flourish, not simply survive. Once we are outside the Victim Cycle, it becomes much clearer that the world isn't full of dangers ready to hurt or kill us. We are not hindering but actually helping ourselves and each other grow in unimaginable ways.

The mainstream blame-based narrative is strong, suggesting we need to be constantly alert and that suffering helps us grow. No pain, no gain, as they say. I have been practicing martial arts and weight training since an early age. I know there are many benefits that come with a certain level of stress and pain. My philosophy isn't about everything being easy and stress-free; it is about becoming aware that there are different types of stress. When it is fueled by blame, victimhood, and fear, we get used to our life being a survival parable about hardship, struggle, and suffering.

But there is another way.

Wired to Learn

The idea that survival, or the ability to live in spite of hardship, is baked into our very DNA is often touted as a good thing. Humans can survive anything if we put our mind to it, we are told. This is often the source of many inspirational movies and documentaries. We love stories where people live through the most extreme of situations. We are told that our survival fight-or-flight instinct can save us when a lion jumps out of the bushes.

The result of this belief, however, is that we have come to think the goal of life is simply to cope and overcome all the pain and suffering that the world will inevitably throw at us. By accepting that we are hardwired for survival, we unknowingly commit ourselves to a life sentence within the Victim Cycle with no option for release. This groupthink puts us in a state of constant fear, where we look to protect ourselves from that "lion" that might attack us at any moment.

It is a real possibility that hardship, struggle, and suffering are symptoms of our blame addiction rather than a built-in requirement of being human. If this is the case, then we are not hardwired for survival. In fact, we are hardwired to learn.

I offer this because I don't see blame play out in any other part of nature. A forest doesn't blame the arsonist or the lightning strike for starting the blaze. And after the burn is extinguished, nature starts the regeneration process immediately. This was epitomized for me when I traveled around Tasmania during a massive bush fire. Driving through roads with raging fire on both sides was a heart-pumping experience. It seemed to me that nothing could come back from such devastation. However, on my return trip two weeks later, I was amazed to find bright green shoots emerging from the scorched tree trunks.

As far as I can see, blame is a uniquely human trait. A dog can certainly remember its abuser and can smell danger and behave in a way to avoid future pain. But Fido will bounce back brighter than before when he is rescued and given the love he craves. Dogs heal so quickly because they don't play the Blame Game. We have the same potential. We simply have to realize at some point that like these radiant green shoots of grass emerging through seemingly impossible odds, our self-honesty is relentlessly pushing through whatever blame- and control-based barriers we place in front of it.

We are always learning about ourselves. The sailors of old who died from scurvy may have believed they were struggling to survive on the high seas. However, they eventually learned their symptoms were actually a message from their bodies. They didn't need to push through the pain and make it to see another day. They just needed some vitamin C. They learned to bring citrus with them on their journeys, and the symptoms disappeared. By listening in a different way, they continued to flourish and ventured farther than they ever had before.

When we search for solutions without the need to find fault, we can effortlessly, honestly, and profoundly self-heal. It's amazing what is possible when, instead of accepting the struggling-to-survive narrative, we instead lean into our hard-wiring to learn. However, this is the important point—what are we learning?

Expert Liars

For thousands of years, we have learned how to become better at blaming, being a victim, and lying to ourselves and others. It can feel uncomfortable to have this realization. It isn't always a conscious process. Often it is just that we are not telling the whole truth.

A client came to me for help with her repetitive strain injury (RSI). This condition involved painful tingling in her hands and wrists. She had been clinically diagnosed and given advice on how to stretch her fingers and make her workstation more ergonomic. But unknowingly, she learned to become better at blaming. This brought short-term relief, but by the time she saw me, even the pharmaceutical painkillers and therapeutic straps were no longer working.

One of the ways I helped my client heal herself was by explaining that if her pain was really caused directly by repetitive movement, then all secretaries, hairdressers, and musicians would have identical RSI symptoms. So why don't they? Because it isn't the repetitive actions themselves that create pain. The symptoms depend on our honest emotional state while we are doing the movements. And I stressed the *honest* part. The fake positive mental attitude we have accepted has helped us become expert liars. Constantly trying to convince ourselves and others we feel different to what we honestly feel is lying. Just ask anyone how they are doing to see how prolific and reflexive it is to lie; inevitably they'll say, "I am good," "I'm fine," "I am doing well." We often lie to ourselves about how we truly feel, to a point where the world is experiencing a pandemic of dishonesty.

My client had managed to put on a brave face for years. She didn't enjoy her work and was having relationship issues at home. She was so used to sweeping her honest emotions and thoughts under the rug, she became numb to just how much physical tension she carried. Her rock-hard shoulders and stiff fingers had become her new normal. Her mind and body had been talking to her for a long time, but she waited until the pain got excruciating before she finally took notice.

My client attempted to ignore and control her symptoms by any means possible. However, after she switched to an attitude of getting more honest with herself, she opened up to consider new possibilities for what the pain might be telling her. She had been feeling broody for a while, but brushed these feelings off, telling herself it was just because she recently became an auntie. When in reality it played on her mind more than she let on to her husband. It might sound unbelievable at this point as you are only a few chapters in, but it was this honest moment as well as many others that helped her RSI symptoms disappear.

Suffice to say, her symptoms had served their purpose of letting her know she wasn't being honest with herself.

No More Sympathy

Blaming your pain on a person or situation is like putting duct tape on a deep wound. Sure, it acts as a great visual aid so you don't see what's going on under the surface. And, yes, it can definitely keep things together. But it won't stop the infection.

At some point, it becomes too painful to ignore. At which point, we often start looking for people to give us sympathy, which is a common way to feed our addiction.

Eventually, just like the barman will stop giving you alcohol when the bar is no longer holding you up, the people helping you receive your blame fix will tire out, leaving you to deal with the resulting pain all by yourself. This is how all victim-based stories end because blame leads to conflict, avoidance, and finally separation. Victimhood can only last so long in other people's eyes before they stop caring and want to get away. Eventually, no amount of pain will be enough to elicit the sympathy or assistance a victim craves.

I once taught a workshop on this, and before we had ventured into the ins and outs of blame, a man in the group raised his hand high, stuck out his chest, and said, "You're wrong! Some people really *are* horrible, and there are innocent victims in the world. Sometimes bad things happen to good people." Before I could clarify what I was saying, he proceeded to tell the room how he'd been totally wronged by his physically abusive father. The group was extremely moved by his recounting of the trauma he had endured. One woman even got up to hug him. Full of empathy for what this man had gone through, I saw this as a great healing opportunity for him and everyone. I asked if he had another story and he quickly obliged. With newfound energy, he launched into a recounting of his experiences with an abusive gym teacher in school. Again, the workshop teared up right along with him. Afterward, I asked, "Do you have any more?" And once again, he charged out of the gates, talking about his abusive ex-wife who took all his money.

As he started a fourth story, about how he'd been treated unfairly by his dishonest business partner, the energy changed in the room. The other workshop participants were less enthusiastic with their displays of sympathy. Nobody was tearing up anymore. The participant who had hugged him the first time offered some constructive criticism based on her own observation, not what we had covered in the workshop. "You are constantly blaming others for what happens in your life," she said. "Can you see how you are taking no responsibility and why abuse and drama gravitate to you? It seems like you are the one who needs to heal." It sounded harsh, because the man had experienced some extreme events. But after four stories with the same theme, everyone could see what needed addressing. He couldn't see it for himself because he was used to getting his blame "high" from others listening to these victim-based stories.

With any addiction, we need to constantly escalate the dosage to receive the same effect. It is why the Blame Game may work in the short term, but it isn't a long-term solution. When we're caught in the Victim Cycle, we focus on honing our denial and seeking self-control rather than self-healing.

You might have heard the parable about the night patrol officer who saw a disheveled, drunken man intently searching the ground underneath a lamppost for his lost keys. The officer asked whether he was certain he lost his keys in this spot, to which the man replied, "No, I lost them somewhere across the street, but the light is better over here."

The groupthink opinion is "bright," so we naturally turn to blame to explain our pain. And we use control-based methods to heal and solve our problems. But what if the "keys" are somewhere different? What if the answer to our problems is whispering from the dark? Maybe all we have to do is something different from what we have always done.

CHAPTER 5

Blame Blinkers

"What do you mean 'blinkers'?" my American editor asked me. "You mean 'blinders,' the contraption you put on horses to impede their peripheral vision. Blinkers are on your car indicating you are turning." Smiling, I said, "Oh, we call them blinkers. And on our car, we call those 'indicators.'"

We laughed, as it demonstrated how you can be thinking you are talking about the same thing but nothing could be further from the truth. I told him a story about when I was at dinner with my American friends and they were talking about an upcoming wedding they were all going to. One of the guys said, "I think we should all wear suspenders...what do you think?"

I laughed, thinking he was joking. "What's so funny?" my friend asked.

"You're going to wear lingerie at your friend's wedding?"

Blame Blinkers

After they explained what they were actually going to wear, it was even funnier. "Oh, you mean braces, what you use to hold up your trousers! That's what we call them in the UK."

"But aren't braces what you put on your teeth?"

For the next thirty minutes we laughed about the differences in our seemingly identical language; pants vs. trousers, condom vs. rubber, buttocks vs. fanny.

Eventually my editor and I settled on blinkers, as I am from the UK.

Even though it was a humorous way of illustrating that not all is as it may seem, it also opens the door of possibility that this is happening much more than we might realize. Maybe life was simpler before language was invented. Maybe we had telepathic abilities where we couldn't hide our self-honesty and had no desire to be dishonest with ourselves or others. It wasn't a thing. But since we have language, it is a good time to get clear about what the impact is when we use certain words and concepts. Otherwise, we are walking around with blinkers on without realizing it.

I mentioned in the previous chapter that I believe the reason for Arnold Schwarzenegger's success is not solely due to his superhuman ability of self-control and determination. It had more to do with him following his unique purpose. He found meaning, as psychiatrist and Holocaust survivor Viktor Frankl would say. As a consequence, Arnold—and indeed Viktor—never survived life; they flourished just like a great redwood that knows it is going to be a great redwood. There is no doubt. They didn't have to convince themselves they were going to survive Auschwitz or become a global superstar—they didn't rely on fake positivity or optimism—they knew.

As amazing as these "true-life survival" and underdog stories are, what is the underlying mindset that is being perpetuated? It is the same one over and over again—get better at finding ways to control your mind, body, and life.

Maybe when they were going through their challenging times, they were not primarily in this survival control-based mentality, but they were, in fact, temporarily living outside of the Victim Cycle. They didn't accept their fate like others did. Their blame blinkers were off, and they were flourishing by being open to alternative possibilities. In contrast, the people who don't make it past these extreme situations are the ones in the victim mindset who bought into the idea that they have to survive. As a result, they are fearful and desperate to escape from their pain. This was their primary focus. So instead of looking for other options, they were fixated on blaming someone or something for their situation. Their anger and need for revenge ate them up inside.

Viktor Frankl is regarded as a Holocaust survivor. It is suggested that he was proactive and used his power to choose his response to the extreme conditions while in the Nazi concentration camps. Viktor himself said, "Everything can be taken from a man but one thing: the last of the human freedoms—to choose one's attitude in any given set of circumstances, to choose one's own way." Many influential people agree with this principle. One of the most famous is Stephen Covey, who wrote *The 7 Habits of Highly Effective People*. He said, "Highly effective people recognize responsibility. They do not blame circumstances, conditions, or conditioning for their behavior. Their behavior is a product of their own conscious choice..." These sentiments sound empowering. And they are when we only look at them superficially. They encourage us to not be a victim of circumstances and to stop blaming other people or events for any so-called negative situations. It sounds like the same message I am offering. However, it is actually as different as braces and suspenders.

Dividing our experiences and emotions into rigid opposites of negative and positive, while thinking we have a conscious choice over our decisions and emotional state, makes sense as it echoes what many wisdom-keepers have said before Viktor and Stephen. Due to this worldview having a well-respected lineage, it has remained unquestioned, not realizing it feeds the survival narrative that our mind, brain, and body are malfunctioning and holding us back. It perpetuates the notion they must be defeated, beaten, and controlled for us to win whatever battle life throws at us tomorrow. It leads us to think blame and the feelings of victimhood, shame, guilt, and anger are like a light switch you can turn on and off at will. However, this becomes a game of peekaboo—it is just an illusion that something has disappeared.

Viktor did something extraordinary. He left the Nazi concentration camps alive when the vast majority didn't. And by all sense of purposes, he was healthy compared to his fellow prisoners. Arnold, the Austrian-born boy who became governor of California, has an astonishing story where he also overcame seemingly impossible hurdles. They both attribute a large part of their success to self-control but also to visualizing what they wanted. For Viktor, it was the deep love of his wife and lecturing to his psychology students. For Arnold, he mentally pictured himself as the champion posing on stage. They both concluded it was their ability to choose their response rather than fall prey to their innate reactions. They went on to promote the virtues of attaining long-term self-control.

It is a confusing message that has left many disappointed and frustrated after attempting to do the same thing. If control and visualization worked as a long-term solution for the masses, then everyone would be who they consciously want to be. This is the crux of the issue. What we become and attain is based on our deep self-honesty, and this is often in conflict with the fake positive wish list we consciously think we want. Both Viktor and Arnold brought to life what they honestly wanted. They used control, but it wasn't their saving grace. Control and survival are not where our focus needs to be if the goal is reaching honest long-term happiness and freedom while attaining new levels of performance and potential.

A Fresh Perspective

I can see one of the reasons depression and suicide are on the rise all around the world is because we have accepted this control- and survival-based narrative. It is stressful and exhausting making our way around the Victim Cycle with blinkers on (again, that's blinders for my American readers) while thinking the idea is to constantly look for new ways to control and defeat certain human reactions that are supposedly holding us back. It's another theory and approach that feeds our blame addiction and makes fear our constant companion. Our primary motivation turns to safety. We put up boundaries to create an environment that limits the chances of anything happening that we would perceive as bad, negative, or wrong.

Thinking that control is the answer to creating a safe existence is a life strategy fraught with blame and victimhood. It stifles joy, adventure, creativity, curiosity, and innovation. It feeds the idea that we can solve our growing fear, shame, and guilt by simply choosing to turn a perceived negative into a positive. It might take training like any muscle, we are told, but with practice we too can have the superpower to be positive and happy all the time. We too can make the right choices and minimize the wrong ones. The strobing effect that results from this black-and-white thinking is exhausting. Jumping from blaming experiences as rigidly negative, positive, right, wrong, good, bad becomes disorientating, especially in a world full of subjectivity and multiculturalism. Being in this mindset all day is turning our blame blinkers inward, narrowing our scope even further. Righteousness sets in, creating room for conflict and mental and physical illness to increase.

It isn't long before we assume life wants to hold us back at any opportunity, believing there are only so many potential partners, dream jobs, and idyllic places to live happy, fulfilled, and successful lives. We remain in us-versus-them mode, entrenched in the mindset that we must constantly fight to gain control of our emotions. We prepare ourselves to battle others for scarce resources and then protect what we have to the death—like a dragon standing over a treasure chest. The issue is that this survival mindset isn't sustainable. It not only requires an enormous amount of energy to maintain, it has us missing opportunities and seeing threats where they don't exist.

"Denis," many clients plead, "just tell me what to do the next time my daughter screams at me." These requests come from a place of desperation. They are the words of someone who feels they have tried everything and nothing has worked. In reality, however, they haven't tried "everything." All they have done is try many different ways to control and conquer themselves, others, or the situation. Because they are operating from a victim mindset, they can't think of any other possibilities.

Playing the Blame Game narrows our focus so that we can only foresee two possible outcomes: positive or negative, helpful or not. It is a bit like those cartoons where someone has an angel on one shoulder and a devil on the other, each vying for our attention. Will we do the right or wrong thing? When we adopt this rigidly black-and-white narrow focus, we unconsciously apply it to every experience. After being a victim for an extended time, everything becomes a matter of good versus evil, and we miss all the color of possibility that is available in any given moment.

Accepting this narrow-focused paradigm results in closed-mindedness. It is commonly seen as an insult to be called ignorant or closed-minded, which is why most of us view ourselves as very open-minded. But is this really true? Are you prepared to listen to a Republican or conservative challenge your ardent beliefs when you are on the opposing side of the table? Are you happy to learn from a vegan about the side effects of eating excessive red meat as you chow down on your succulent steak? Would you be open to listening to a so-called conspiracy theorist inform you of their latest thoughts about government secret agendas?

Classing ourselves as open-minded when we are not paradoxically leads us to do very little about opening our minds any further. We prefer to stay away from certain people because we blame them for being stupid or crazy, not realizing the scientists, inventors, and innovators we admire today were referred to in the same way not long ago. Our blame addiction is being constantly fed while we simultaneously divide our experiences into whether something is rigidly good or bad, possible or not. We don't realize that much of the time when we are in this righteous mindset, we are also in a state of incomplete information, awareness, or wisdom.

We accuse the vegan of being a pain in the ass, only to become plant-based a year later when a doctor's advice changes our mind. Ten years of anger toward your brother can disappear when you find out he didn't do what you thought he did. As much as you know the untold benefits that come with being more open-minded, can you honestly say you are blinker-free in *all* situations with *all* people *all* the time?

Many people aspire to gain the ability to listen, share opinions, and debate ideas without labeling them as right or wrong or accepting them as truth. However, few actually achieve this. Even the ones who consider themselves open-minded can have great poker faces as they masterfully hide their honest feelings when they listen to others. The cool, calm, and measured exterior of these in-control individuals can hide a righteousness or irritation that makes subtle appearances in their interactions.

I am not saying we should sit back and let all the abuses in the world pass us by. I am also not saying the answer is to suddenly reveal all our honest emotions that we have spent a lifetime controlling. I am saying one of the most effective strategies we have for helping ourselves and others create a life devoid of abuse is to heal from our blame addiction. This whole book is here to offer an approach to achieve that goal. An important part of this philosophy is to train our perception muscle. This is how we pry our minds open so we feel comfortable walking around without blame blinkers on, feeling confident to apply a fresh perspective to each situation we encounter.

Seeing With One Eye Open

Imagine you are driving down a lonely country road when... *bam!* Out of nowhere, you hit a dog. In your rearview mirror you can see the poor animal, bloody, lying on the pavement, still alive, panting, eyes rolling in agony and fear. Do you stop, or do you keep driving?

What is the right and kind thing to do?

If you're like many of my clients, you might immediately and righteously respond with something like, "Of course I would stop, Denis, I'm not a monster!" It seems obvious that the good, kind, and caring response would be tending to the injured animal or putting it out of its misery. But what if it was midnight and you had never been on this country road before? What if you also had your six-month-old baby in the car with you? What if you were on your way to tend to your teenage daughter who had just called with an emergency? Would it make a difference what you did if you had no phone reception or if you were vegan or a butcher? Scared of dogs or not?

What would the good, kind, and caring response be in these situations?

I use moral dilemmas as a way to open our minds to other possibilities. These hypotheticals illustrate that not is all as it may seem in any given moment. We commonly have a tolerance threshold, and when this point is crossed, we can act in hypocritical ways and do things that go against our ardent beliefs, morals, and values. We are experts at using creative mental gymnastics to justify these types of opposing actions. However, going against what we preach as "right" can produce subtle feelings of guilt and shame, regardless of how convincingly we rationalize our actions. In time, this internal conflict contributes to mental and physical stress and illness.

Some people hearing the dog scenario have assured me that no matter what the extenuating circumstances look like, tending to the animal is always the "right" and "kind" thing to do. This is certainly a commendable stance, and over a dinner table these individuals would be considered caring and kind, especially if another guest admitted they would put their foot down and speed off. However, we may need to take into account what heavyweight champion boxer Mike Tyson famously said: "Everybody has a plan until they get punched in the mouth." We can talk a good game and be rigid and righteous in our projections, but when the unexpected happens we take on a very different persona and attitude. One minute we are blaming the other person for being selfish and mean, only to quickly change our mind and transfer the blame onto ourselves for "jumping to conclusions."

Hypocrisy is rampant in our world today because it is a symptom of our growing addiction to blame.

Perhaps you pride yourself on sticking to your morals and would stop for the wounded dog *no matter what*, even with your sick baby in the back seat, as you rush to help your stranded teenage daughter, and the massive tornado whips through the canyon, heading straight toward your car. But if you do stop under these circumstances, are you prepared to take responsibility for your part in anything that happens? Or will you later blame the unexpected severity of the weather that you couldn't control?

It might sound like I am encouraging you to drive on, but that's not what I'm getting at. I am ramping up the scenario to illustrate the point that we are constantly walking a fine line between classing ourselves as a victim or empowered. With one extra piece of information, our ardent stance can completely change. Blaming someone for being "foolhardy" is easy. But in hindsight, or with a different perspective, you might describe them as a "hero" if they ended up saving lives. This is why stopping is very much a viable option, along with many other possibilities.

The question is, in your daily life, are you honing your existing skill of seeing the world as a black-and-white movie or one that is full of 8K technicolor possibilities?

Most of us, when considering this type of moral dilemma, quickly jump to choosing a side: stop or don't stop. We don't like to think that maybe there is no absolute answer. We fail to consider the possibility that the answer is *always* conditional. We reactively designate a good versus bad way to act, and we ignore all the messy factors that could push the morality of our actions into a gray area.

When we immediately dichotomize a situation into helpful versus unhelpful, we are perpetually looking at the world with one eye closed. Yes, we can still see, but what are we missing on the periphery?

Seeing the World as 0s and 1s

We have all grown up watching detective films, shows, and cartoons. One of my favorite scenes of all time is from the 1976 film *The Pink Panther Strikes Again*. It is the moment where Inspector Clouseau hilariously bumbles around, interrogating his suspects. He jumps to new conclusions each time he finds out new information. Other detectives are less black and white when investigating a case. They are open and curious to discover more information before making their judgment at the big reveal.

We have created a way of rationalizing, innovating, and constructing machines based on this binary 0 and 1 model. It works when we are building machines and computers. However, humans are neither, and in life the truth is often relative.

I am not advocating moral relativism and suggesting "to each their own" or "when in Rome, do as the Romans do." And I am definitely not saying we should go morally bankrupt and become devoid of any value system. Rather, I'm demonstrating that our rigid attachment to dichotomies is what contributes to the issues that we are looking to change in our personal lives and in the world at large. This need to divide and pick a side is rooted in our blame addiction.

Many people believe it is judgment that causes so much pain and discomfort. We often hear, "Don't judge me!" or "You are being so judgmental right now." It has got a reputation for being a troublemaker. But actually, do you know what the definition of "judgment" is? Very few people have thought about it. I know I just accepted the mainstream opinion that it was bad and we should do it less. If it was such a negative space to be in, then why does it have synonyms that most people would see as compliments, like "common sense," "intelligence," "knowledge," "wisdom," and "astuteness"?

To judge is to make a definitive decision based on all the information that is available. It is what a judge in a courtroom or a CEO in a boardroom does every day. What we can actually feel is the blame being thrown around—"Don't blame me!" or "You are being so blamey right now." We have demonized "judging," which is something we need to do every day, and we need to get better at it—not fear it. The reason many people don't like making decisions is because we have accepted this narrow view of what judgment means. But again, it means discernment, to go beyond what is on the surface to make considered decisions.

Making judgment calls is something we do all day, depending on what is happening in the moment. The issue is, we use past experience to determine a risk analysis about what will happen now and in the future, not realizing all our past evidence is steeped in blame. It is why we keep co-creating the same experiences. We think we are making different choices, but they are all emanating from the same foundation ladened with blame, victimhood, fear, and a need for control. The more we ignore training our creativity and perception muscle, the more it atrophies and our mind closes down.

The thing to do in any situation is complex and multifaceted. A confident leader will be open to debate and make a definitive decision based on all the information available to them. They will continue to be open to changing circumstances and ready to make another judgment call. The rest of nature follows this approach. Nature doesn't dichotomize in a rigid way, so why do we? We are part of the same ecosystem here on Earth. Nature constantly adapts and flourishes when left to its own devices. There is no blame or victimhood in nature. In fact, when nature is being controlled by the rigid parameters that humans regularly impose, it decays. Counterintuitively, humans would also flourish, and not fall into anarchy, if we learned from what nature does so naturally. It is blame and the feelings of victimhood and fear that lead to anarchy, not the lack of rules and structure.

It is easy to get righteous about actions like using child labor in sweatshops, torturing another human to get sensitive intel, mutilating animals for medical research, or accepting collateral damage of women and children in a so-called holy war. But these events are applauded or ignored every day around the world. Often, the people who would condemn an act under one set of circumstances are in favor of the same act when the context changes. We are against children being made to work, but we love our new phone. We are against animal cruelty, but that burger was delicious. We are against murder, but proud of our sons and daughters fighting for their country.

As a personal trainer, I would beat myself up for having a pizza when I spent the day telling my clients to stay away from carbs. Of course, I learned to rationalize my way out of the guilt. I could gorge on an extra-large treat because I worked out for two hours and they didn't. Telling your teenage son to stop smoking while you convince yourself that you only smoke when you go out with the boys is easy. Laying a thick guilt trip on your eight-year-old for not eating their broccoli is seen as good parenting. But how do you answer the question, "Daddy why don't you eat broccoli?"

Being in this hypocritical space is one leading reason why we are so exhausted. We are in a constant state of denial. Lying to ourselves and others takes a lot of energy. The more we blame, the more righteous we become. The doors of possibility remain closed when there are so many to open. It is a perpetuating cycle that leads to us co-create ever more extreme levels of conflict and drama, as this is how we get the majority of our blame fixes. It is why we think things can't go well for too long and why we think life would be boring if we didn't have drama.

Many people can't relax and enjoy the moments when life is going well because they start to think that shit will hit the fan soon. But actually, all that is happening is that we haven't had our blame fix for a while, so we unconsciously go looking for it.

In order to make our blame fix easier, we box and label people together. It gives us a bigger target to point our fingers at.

CHAPTER 6

Attached to a Label

In my early twenties, I received an important lesson on the power of labels. During a night out with a friend and my then girlfriend, I couldn't believe how they ganged up on me. I had very thick skin, of course, after years of diligently practicing the art of denial and locking my true feelings away. So it took a lot of poking the bear before the beast finally revealed itself. As the evening unfolded, however, the alcohol loosened up my stoic self-control, allowing the bubbling anger to build into a dramatic crescendo. The silent battle in my head changed the energy at the table. My girlfriend felt it first. Of course she did, as all the blame was silently directed at her.

"Are you okay, Den?" she asked.

"Why are you trying to make me look stupid?" I complained.

Her denials couldn't penetrate my defenses. I confidently turned to my loyal best friend for support and confirmation of her outrageous and disrespectful behavior. But it didn't arrive.

He defended her, saying she was being funny. At that point, the beast was out.

"Chill out, let it go," he shrugged. "Stop being overly sensitive." But this advice had an effect similar to pouring gasoline on a bonfire. Over the past hour I had already implemented the first option that blame left me with: I tried to suck it up and put on a brave face. Now that had run its course, it was time for option two. Separation—I stormed out of the bar.

There are many moving parts that keep us in the Victim Cycle that make us categorize a certain event as rigidly good or bad. Labels play a huge factor as each one comes with a conscious and unconscious list of how they should and shouldn't behave. My friend and I jousted for the best one-liners at each other's expense all evening, and I had no problem with that. The banter was funny when it came from him. But somehow it felt different when similar jabs came from my girlfriend. They felt like uppercuts into the solar plexus. I didn't realize then that the attachments I had to these labels dramatically influenced my perceptions of their behavior.

It is not that labels are the problem. They certainly help us navigate our daily interactions. There are etiquette and protocols to be aware of. We do sometimes need to treat our boss differently than we treat our romantic partner. However, when we have an attachment to how that label should and shouldn't behave, we are unknowingly giving ourselves an opportunity to be a victim. We are blaming them (or ourselves) for not behaving in the right, ideal, or perfect way. But are there such ideals that can be applied to all people at all times? After spending three years studying East Asian Studies at university where I did a deep dive into the cultures and business practices of China, Japan, North and South Korea, I became very aware how differently we all see the world. It is easy to make rigid assertions in how someone should behave or even be brought up, but they can fall apart when you apply them to another culture, environment, or circumstance.

Earlier in my business career, I used to treat others in radically different ways based on their professional labels. I would talk to someone for twenty minutes at a networking event, thinking how amazing and wonderful they were. Then all those complimentary feelings would vanish upon hearing that what they did for a living couldn't benefit me in some way. That deep feeling of connection and synergy immediately turned into a comical production of excuses to leave. On the other hand, if their label matched my professional goals or moral standing, I would launch into an impressive performance of sucking up.

Labels are powerful. One piece of information or one experience can change everything. But again, labels and the expectation we place on them are not the enemy; it is the attachment (blame) to how they should behave that creates closed-mindedness, stress, and conflict.

One client told me how he changed his opinion of lawyers after a drawn-out and painful divorce. Before this experience, he used to love chatting with them. He found them clever, driven, and well-connected. After the divorce, however, he could never see them in the same light again. He blamed them for his unhappiness, and it created the attachment that lawyers are now manipulative, mean, and the enemy.

It is easy to get attached and group people and things together under one umbrella. All police are the same. All snakes are dangerous. All bankers are evil. However, as Kevin Richardson, the lion whisperer, mentioned in his book, *Part of the Pride*, "Conventional wisdom, among lion keepers, I later learned, was that one should never trust a lion with clear eyes. Like a lot of things people told me about lions over the years to come, and conventional wisdom in general, that little gem turned out to be bullshit...I'd already broken all these rules before I even knew they existed."

It is why, when it comes to my labels and the labels of others, instead of being attached to how they should behave, I have *preference*.

I now have preferences for how my lawyer, friend, girlfriend, or client behaves, in the same way I do when I see my mother, nieces, or sister. I have a preference for how I will turn up as a son, brother, and friend. But because I have gone through the honest healing process detailed in this book, the attachment (blame) is naturally no longer there. We are free to live inside or outside the societal ideals or traditions that exist. It creates space for you to expand and freedom to be who you honestly are.

I know my girlfriend and I are different than who we were yesterday, as are my business partner, accountant, and client. It is no different than any other aspect of nature. Even the oldest tree in the world—a Great Basin bristlecone pine, which is said to be around five thousand years old—is different every day in some way. So every time I communicate with anyone, it will be *for the first time*. Because I am now fully aware that change is a constant, there is naturally no attachment or acceptance of what was, or what I think should be. There is just openness to be curious and explore the new us.

If the people in my life don't match my preference, my instant reaction is no longer disappointment, frustration, and anger. I am now empathetic and curious, meaning I am open to the many other possibilities as to what might be happening. They might be sick or have some news they are not sharing. They might be planning a surprise party and can't tell me. A pet might have just passed away. So many reasons could be playing out as to why they are behaving differently than what I am used to.

Again, it comes down to whether we are prepared to put in the work to train our creative and perception muscles so we are open enough to entertain all the possibilities that are available. Otherwise, we will continue to interact with the "labels" in our life and not the actual people behind them.

The Power of a Label

We can perhaps best see the power of labels at play when it comes to categorizing people. We love to make sweeping generalizations, declaring, "My wife's always doing things like this!" or "My husband will never change." We use personality tests to group our colleagues, zodiac signs to index our lovers, and ethnic backgrounds to classify strangers.

In a relatively short period of time, a stranger can become a friend, girlfriend, fiancée, wife, and mother of your child. That could be a change of six labels in a twelve-month period. Is it possible that as the label changes so does the attachment to how that label should and shouldn't behave? Maybe. You might be proud of your friend for getting attention from men by dancing drunk on the table, but how do you feel if she does the same thing the next day when she becomes your girlfriend?

Have you ever heard someone say, "I don't understand; it was like he changed overnight after we got married"? Change can happen quickly while we are consciously or unconsciously attached to what a label represents. A client once told me how caring and supportive her fiancé was. For the previous two years he was so encouraging about a new business venture she was planning. However, during the honeymoon he made it abundantly clear that he wanted her to be a stay-at-home mother to look after the big family they were going to have.

The reality is that all the while we are addicted to blame we change when we come into contact with a label whether we are aware of it or not. Many people have assured me this is not the case, and they pride themselves on treating everyone the same. It is a commendable stance, but is it true? Or are they just really good at controlling their honest feelings and prejudices?

One of my clients showcased this perfectly. She was a very high-powered City of London trader. She had it all together, and it took a lot to faze her. However, with everyone's consent I arranged for a celebrity client of mine to briefly meet her, as he was her idol. It was amazing to see how cool she was up to the very minute she saw him. It was especially interesting because many people had just walked past him without knowing who he was. His label and what he represented is what she responded to as she turned into a shy giggling teenager.

When we change from boyfriend to husband, or employee to manager, we update our behavior to match what we *think* the new label should and shouldn't be based on our own personal ideals and that of others and society.

It can get complicated, as not everyone perceives the label in the same way. Thus, we add an additional layer of complexity. People are regularly categorized as a good or bad version of their label. We have good dads versus bad ones, exceptional girlfriends versus crummy ones, and great bosses versus terrible ones. One person might get promoted and go on a power trip while another might experience a humbling effect due to the added responsibility.

I can now see how I constantly held people in a fixed paradigm and how much stress this was causing in my life. I realized that so many of my issues and arguments were not with the people themselves, or their behaviors, but with my attachment to what their label should and shouldn't act like. I would become upset if the person didn't match what I thought was respectful, appropriate, and kind behavior. I was being naive to think my rigid view was universal for all people in all situations in all cultures. Life is multifaceted, multicultural, and multidimensional for a reason. We can see so many more options when we are not wearing our blame goggles. We become curious rather than running around and accusing everyone of being the prime suspect for our unhappiness.

Labels are everywhere, and we need them to converse. We label everything from weather and dog breeds to cities and career choices. Countries are first, second, or third world. Schools are public or private. Paintings are impressionistic or postmodern.

It's not that labels are the problem (actually, to label labels as bad would be a blame-based response). However, for honest healing to take place it is helpful to become aware of our attachment to our labels. Friends and best friends can behave in the same way, but we might have different rules for each. For example, if a friend cancels on coming to our birthday party at the last minute, we might be less upset than if a best friend did the same, especially if they both had the same excuse. The action was the same but the label was different. We might even downgrade the best friend to the status of a friend because they didn't behave how a best friend should. As we will explore in much more detail in later chapters, we do this all the while not realizing our addiction to blame and the *self-honesty* it hides is what needs addressing, not what our friend or best friend did or didn't do.

It is worth reiterating: the majority of our arguments are with the labels in our lives, not the people behind the labels and their actions. When I started to become aware of this, I would ask myself a simple question when I was ready to self-reflect on an argument I'd had with my girlfriend. I would ask, "Would I talk to my mother, sister, friend, or boss like that if they did the same thing?" The answer was invariably a no, and it indicated I was angry with my attachment to the label of girlfriend and not her actual behavior.

Since I was used to interacting with labels rather than the people behind them, I went about life collecting as many labels for myself as I could. It wasn't just family or professional labels I took on. No, I sought out psychological ones too, like "dyslexia," "fear of abandonment," and "commitment issues." It felt good to get a new label. Why? Because it was unknowingly another way of getting my blame fix. I can't pass exams because of my dyslexia. I can't stay in a relationship because of my commitment issues. None of which were true.

Many modern psychological diagnoses—narcissist, egotistical, bipolar, or perfectionist—are taken as a license for us to blame ourselves or others and use them as excuses. We might think that labels that come with certain experiences in our past were responsible for our current struggles. It's acceptable to say things like, "Your father left your mother when you were only five, so that's why you have abandonment issues." We use this type of narrative as a way to excuse our lack of intimate relationships. Or you conclude, "My mother was stressed when I was a baby, so I have an anxiety disorder and scare off friends." Or, "My parents did everything for me when I was younger, so I don't feel I can do anything for myself now." Developmental psychology is great if you want to find out why people do what they do so you can sell to them more effectively or you need to predict the behavior of a serial killer. Unpacking the human psyche in this respect can be helpful. But when it comes to honestly healing and being honestly happy, the more labels we collect and become attached to, the more we are confusing a healing process that is designed to be simple.

We become so attached to our long-standing labels and the victim-based narratives surrounding them that we have difficulty seeing any alternative perspectives. We grow attached to and focus on blame-based stories that are familiar, and this is another way we stay in the Victim Cycle. It teaches us to throw blame bombs at our parents for not bringing us up based on a rigid set of ideals. But where did those ideals come from? What is the perfect upbringing we think we missed out on? When I ask my clients these questions, they often don't have an answer. Like myself many years ago, they have gotten so used to casting a huge net of blame, they haven't taken the time to see what they actually caught. It wasn't evidence they were right about missing out as a child; it was a haul of decaying rubbish. It leads us to create a life based on the lies we tell ourselves.

Our ideals come from religions, traditions, TV shows, films, Disney, and what we think other children had that we didn't. And these ideals are different all over the world. So again, what is the ideal upbringing we believe we missed out on? It isn't a fact that abused children go on to abuse others. Or that children who are surrounded by opulence and the best education go on to be model citizens. The human experience is infinitely complex, but with that said, it is magically simple when you explore the possibility everything might be unfolding to help you.

As I said to a client, "You don't know who your mum or dad actually are." I was leading into the idea that they have only ever interacted with the labels. Every conversation has been through the lens of what a good and bad parent is. It is the same with siblings and children. We grow up reacting to each other's label. A beautiful and magical thing can happen with these relationships when we get to finally know who is behind the label.

Accepting a Label

A client wanted to heal from his so-called "ten-year battle with arthritis." When I suggested his war-based description and acceptance of his label was unknowingly keeping him in a state of pain, his defenses shot up and he fiercely rationalized his label like a seasoned lawyer. He quickly launched into a speech about how real his arthritis was, especially for people around his age. He'd received a medical diagnosis, and without that he wouldn't have been able to receive medication to treat his symptoms.

What he was actually convincing me of was how real his pain had been for the past ten years. I assured him I was empathetic to all the pain he had experienced. My goal was to help him become aware of how his acceptance of his label was in fact one of the main reasons he was still in pain a decade later. His acceptance acted like a lock and key, postponing the self-healing process.

I also pointed out that, although he was only fifty-nine, he clung to the assertion that he was "old." This went hand in hand with the arthritis diagnosis. He believed the same narrative that the majority of the world believes: as we age, we degrade, become frail, and get ill. And he was collecting labels along the journey to back up that story. Many of us do exactly the same thing, even though there is evidence all around us to the contrary. There are places around the world called "blue zones," where an unprecedented percentage of people live to over one hundred, all the while staying fit and healthy.

It is common for people to compete for the most extreme label. Talking about their ailments, surgeries, and doctors becomes a way for people to bond. My client was part of this reality. He was evoking a self-fulfilling prophecy. His diagnosis and label were considered incurable. He'd been told it could only be managed, not fully healed, and that the symptoms would progressively get worse. By accepting the diagnosis, he gave all his healing power over to the doctors. He effectively blamed his body for doing something wrong and stopped listening to and seeing his symptoms and pain as the guides that they are. All doors of possibility were slammed shut to him making a full recovery.

Of course, accepting his label and seeing it as a battle was the absolute right path for my client, as he didn't know any other options existed. Doctors or the pharmaceutical industry that trains them are not in the firing line for blame. Once new possibilities become apparent, it is for us to realize that whoever we go to for help are facilitators for us to heal ourselves.

My goal with any client who comes to me with a medical or psychological label is to disrupt their attachment and acceptance of their label and diagnosis. Each label comes with its own set of perceptions about what is possible and how the symptoms might show up over time. The doctors and psychiatrists make diagnoses with their blame blinkers and blame-tinted glasses on. They divide the mind and body into sections, systems, and organs, forgetting that we are an ecosystem working symbiotically together. The allopathic model is a healing system that will keep a blame addict coming back for more, as there is always a more severe label (i.e., a higher "high") to be attained.

When we accept the rigid definitions that come with our labels, we postpone our ability to self-heal, either physically or emotionally.

Many clients come to me with seemingly impossible conditions and can't believe how quickly they see a change in their symptoms when their relationship to the label changes. Their body starts to rejuvenate in ways that leave them thinking the results must be a trick or temporary. Before this, their experience with healing has been slow, arduous, and never complete, especially when they consider themselves as old. Naturally they are applying the blame-based cause-and-effect logic. I have been in pain for ten years, so I will be in more pain for the next ten. It is why so many of my older clients want to die, because the thought of living with their label and dire diagnosis is too much to bear.

Blame is so integrated into our psyche and vocabulary that it takes practice to unearth all the places it is hiding. That includes where it is hiding in our body. I worked with my arthritic client for a year. But his symptom and pain levels went down 95 percent within a few weeks. We mostly worked on his blame-induced anger issues, which showed up as stiffness and "inflammation" in his body. Within a very short time he had rejuvenated his entire mind and body to the point he felt more mentally alert and physically fit than he had been when he was thirty. His doctor couldn't believe how his other long-term "autoimmune" disease had reversed. The transformation was so astonishing, a year later his new doctor was convinced he had been misdiagnosed, as he couldn't fathom how this particular label could ever reverse. It was a great illustration of how narrow-minded and attached some professionals can become to particular labels, and how that victim-based perception is projected for others to accept. Or not.

Labels are undoubtedly helpful. I am not advocating we get rid of them all. Rather, I offer that when we see how our attachment and acceptance of them keeps us in a tight paradigm of possibility, we see our relationship with them change. And as we do, we mentally and physically heal in profound ways, often in time frames that would be regarded as impossible.

Like thinking we are wired for survival or to notice what is negative or wrong, being attached to how labels should behave narrows our focus and generates fear. When we are open to more possibilities, we no longer feel the need to search the streets looking for our next blame hit. The pursuit of control dwindles along with our fear. It can sound too simple. And that is often the issue. We are used to overcomplicating the self-healing process that is designed to be simple and effortless.

Opening Doors of Possibility

When I talk about being attached to labels and how disempowering it is to accept them, it can sound like I am ignoring the severity of the symptoms that led to getting the diagnosis. Of course I am not. I am bringing awareness that regardless of the label, all of the symptoms are indicators we are in our blame addiction. I see it every day with clients. As they proceed along the recovery process, their symptoms lessen and disappear. Meaning the label was always an illusion. Albeit a powerful one. It works this way because the less blame we have running around our mind, body, and life, the more self-honest we naturally become. And this is the key to profound feelings of freedom and happiness.

The issue is, the number of labels we can choose from are rising exponentially. We love to use acronyms like IBS, ADHD, and OCD to label our pain, not realizing they keep us victims because we are blaming the diagnoses for our behavior. We say things like, "I can't go on that camping vacation—I need to be near a toilet to manage my IBS!" or "My ADHD makes it really hard to acquire new skills" or "I can never get anything done because my OCD has me compulsively checking for cracks in the plaster of my office." I hear many times how "these are facts, not excuses. I am not blaming or being a victim. These are the things I have to learn to live with."

I offer clients other possibilities to once again train their perception muscle so they can become free of their label and exit the Victim Cycle they don't realize they are in. I play a game with them, asking for as many possible honest reasons they can come up with that might shine some light on more honest motivations. Perhaps they don't truly want to go camping for their vacation or acquire new skills for a job they hate. Some clients, in a moment of deep self-honesty, have admitted they use their labels to punish their parents by showing them how messed up they are—"Look what you did to me!" Other clients have simply acknowledged they really didn't like their partner's friends and that is why they didn't want to go camping.

We default to blaming our labels to explain our behavior because it's easy. Being honest with ourselves feels strange in a world where hyper-fake positivity is promoted as the best mindset to have. With that said, being self-honest can also be easy; we just have to start the blame-recovery process.

Labels, blame, dichotomies, attachment, and victimhood keep us looping around on the same exhausting rinse cycle. We experience stress, pain, hardship, dishonesty, and disconnection from others. We seek control, narrow our focus, and downplay our honest feelings and dreams. Many people feel stuck without meaning or purpose. These are symptoms of being in the Victim Cycle for an extended period of time. There are opportunities all around us to exit the cycle and be happier, but we just don't see them.

I once used a simple example to express this point to a group I was working with. My friend was visiting and asked to borrow my phone charger. I directed her to the television in the living room where I had a spare.

"It isn't here!" she called to me.

I walked into the living room, only to find her poking around the TV stand with the cable next to her foot.

I asked my group: Why couldn't she see the phone charger, even though she was nearly stepping on it?

Some of their replies were: "She wasn't listening to the instructions," "She was looking the other way," and "She was upset and distracted." All these suggestions could be correct, but I was looking for a specific answer.

I clarified that my friend had an Apple iPhone and asked, "What color cable was she attached to finding?"

"White!" was the general consensus around the room.

At this point I revealed that the charging cable on the floor was blue. In my friend's mind she had an unspoken attachment about the label "iPhone charger"—it must be white. Her mind was so focused on uncovering a white cable cord, she was blind to the alternate option just beneath her toes. This is what fed her blame of me giving her the wrong instructions, coupled with her self-blame of not being able to find it.

There are times when dogged determination, laser focus, and absolute single-mindedness are necessary to complete a task or hone a skill. But there is an argument to say, even when we need to focus in this way, we would benefit from being open at the same time.

The fact is: our blame addiction and the need to control, accept, and play the victim has meant that narrow-mindedness has become our new normal. The fear, shame, guilt, anger, and regret that results mean we are not as open to the many other possibilities available to us in any given experience.

A client once asked me, "I don't understand what you are saying. I don't get it. If I can't blame others, and I can't blame myself—what do I do?"

For most people, they haven't spent one second venturing into the possibility that we could live in a world where playing the Blame Game isn't a normal part of life. However, there is a third possibility...one that enables us to once again remember what powerful self-healing organisms we are.

CHAPTER 7

Creators or Controllers

A common line of thinking is to believe there are people who stop us from getting what we want. Or that our shitty opinion of ourselves is holding us back from enjoying life. Positive psychology, self-development, and philosophical traditions like Buddhism suggest that we can overcome unhealthy relationships and achieve the type of life we truly deserve if we can just master self-control and be positive, set boundaries, cut out toxic people, let go of energy vampires, separate ourselves from our negative thoughts, love ourselves, and manage our abandonment issues. This attitude feels right because it is steeped in blame.

When we think this way, it becomes gradually easier to blame others for stirring up drama, causing pain, and disrespecting our boundaries. The combination of blame and control encourages us to believe the narrative that the innate design of the human is faulty. That we are malfunctioning in some way. That our thoughts and beliefs are holding us back. There are numerous success-oriented events we can attend that promise to show us the latest neuroscience on how to delete, reframe, and rewire our negative thoughts into success-driven positive ones.

Without realizing it, this approach to happiness and success is a reflection that we are in the final stages of our blame addiction. It shows up as separation. I blame my girlfriend, she blames me. It continues until we can't take it anymore and we separate, hoping to never see each other again. We do the same with our thoughts. I blame them, they blame me. We can't take it anymore and do everything we can to shut them up before we just tap out and leave. It is why depression, fear, and suicide are so rampant in our world today, even though we have unrivaled access to the very wisdom that is supposed to help us become happier.

What happens when we no longer accept these pieces of advice? Suddenly we become curious to look behind the curtain to see what is being sold.

It is a very tempting proposition with a great and compelling sales pitch. It has made it easy to accept. The taglines are enticing: "Learn how to free yourself from yourself. Stop self-sabotaging yourself, and you will be rich and happy." It could be an old or new meditation practice to distract yourself from your so-called negative chatter or some form of hypnosis so you can reprogram or separate yourself from these supposedly destructive thoughts altogether.

Neuroscience is used to back this up. We are told our mind focuses more on the negative than the positive. Various mindfulness practices tell us that "you are not your thoughts" and

the negative ones are pointless, unhelpful, and have no purpose whatsoever (apart from holding us back). When we hear
this, it adds credence to the sales pitch that while part of you
doesn't want these thoughts, another part of you does—like
your "pain-body," as popularized by the new age guru Eckhart
Tolle. We are told that the goal is to sever the link between your
thought processes and body. To help with this, an instruction is
given to be more "compassionate" and "surrender" to what is.
But again, why do these sentiments feel right?

They all have a foundation in blame and victimhood.
The promoters are unaware they have an addiction to blame
playing out. If you are so inclined, look up the definitions of
compassion and *surrender*. You might change your mind in
using them again. Not is all as it may seem when you question
the unquestionable and look behind the curtain.

Part of the blame-recovery process is to question everything we have been told. Otherwise, we will continue to blame
news channels, social media, and violent movies for the reason
we behave the way we do. The same blame- and control-based
message is on repeat: Just be mindful that you have unnecessary, useless, and dysfunctional thinking. Your brain is trying
to deceive you. You can't control your thoughts, but you can
control the meaning you assign to them and how you react. So
learn how to reframe and rewire your thoughts and become
the master of your mind (brain). It becomes exhausting to follow these edicts, because they are trying to fix something that
doesn't need fixing. Our fear of doing things wrong becomes
our constant companion under these doctrines. When they
no longer work, more labels like imposter syndrome, anxiety

disorder, and chronic fatigue syndrome are doled out and eagerly accepted.

Is this really how it works? Aren't we just doing the same thing expecting different results? This whole line of thinking leads to the simple conclusion: if we change our thinking, we change our reality. But this is just code for "get better at self-control and rid yourself of negative thoughts and be more positive." We are back to teaching ourselves how to be expert liars and masterful victims.

There is a side effect of this approach to achieving happiness and success. Over time, the more you accept that your mind and body are doing all they can to stand in your way to being happy, feelings of fear, shame, guilt, anger, and regret start to reveal themselves in ever more extreme ways.

We don't need any of these painful side effects when we become aware we are actually creators in life. And our mind and body are seamlessly interconnected and working overtime to help us in every way they can to uncover who we honestly are.

Perfect Design

Have you ever walked around a forest or jungle and thought, *This is a poor design*? It might look chaotic and full of disorder, but something in you, even if you are not a trained horticulturist, knows there is a rhyme and reason for everything that is happening. We become engrossed in the weird and wonderful ways everything works together. At first, we might not understand why a particular type of mushroom or moss is growing or dying in that specific place, but when we look deeper into the microbiome or further up into the canopy, reasons start to reveal themselves.

How is it that we don't look at our mind, brain, body, and life in the same way? Could it be that we no longer feel connected with nature? After years of blaming ourselves, others, and nature for doing things wrong, are we now in the ultimate stage of our blame addiction—separating ourselves from Earth and looking to live on Mars?

Like nature, our mind and body aren't poorly designed. As a symbiotic system, it is a perfect design. We just have to look at it when we don't have our blame attire covering our senses. The mainstream narrative keeps us believing that humans are controllers, not creators. However, the evidence to the contrary is all around us to see. We generate life force energy from being creative and exploring possibility. Just look at the boundless energy and reaction of a baby or young child when they discover something new. Or when they are playing in their imagination. Their energy is infectious. And then look what happens when they are being controlled or they are trying to contain their anger. Our little angel turns into a little Hulk.

Because blame is a human construct not found in other parts of nature, we believe that our symptoms, pains, and self-deprecating thoughts are hinderances and enemies blocking us from reaching happiness. We have been living a lie. When we get curious, we finally see the very thoughts we are told are negative, unnecessary, destructive, or useless are in fact working in weird and wonderful ways to help us. They're signposts, aids, and teachers relentlessly helping us reach new levels of self-honesty so we can achieve more than we think is possible. When we get this, it can be astonishing how quickly these tapes run out. It is like a naughty child getting the attention they want. They are relentless in their goal, and when they are listened to, they calm down. It might take time, and a couple of rounds to get to this point, but when we get better at listening earlier and earlier, peace and harmony are the result.

I understand this viewpoint needs more qualitative and quantitate substance to back up such a claim, and that is what this whole book is here to provide. As one of my very first editors, nearly ten years ago, said, "Denis, your book is going to help so many people...but I have to say it is so counterintuitive!"

Of course, he is right. It is because there are so many extreme events and acts of abuse going on in the world. It leaves us with the obvious conclusion that we really do live in a Marvel movie where good and evil are constantly battling it out. But isn't this just an endless narrative we have heard for thousands of years? Isn't it just a self-fulfilling prophecy we keep perpetuating? It is a circular argument that keeps us victimizing ourselves by asserting we are being bullied or mistreated.

It won't necessarily feel like these painful and incessant thoughts are helping us after decades of being in an MMA fight with them, doing all we can to knock them out or beat them into submission. Because we have been in the Victim Cycle for so long, we have trained ourselves to divide our thoughts into two black-and-white camps: helpful and unhelpful. But maybe more is playing out. Maybe life isn't designed to be diluted down to such rigid extremes. Maybe this is one of the reasons nature is so full of color and diversity.

When does a beautiful flower become an ugly weed and a majestic deer become an irritable pest? Is it when we don't understand what is going on and deem it uncontrollable? How can someone dream of dying while they are asleep and call it a nightmare or bad omen, while another person or culture will regard this as a sign of opportunity and rebirth? How much welcomed motivation do we receive before we claim we are being unfairly bullied?

Our thoughts are not the enemy. Nor is our mind, brain, or body.

Life feels more painful and effortful when we keep following the blame and control approach to life because we are fighting the strongest force in nature—self-honesty. The very thoughts we think are negative are our honest thoughts. And rather than sever them, we need to build a connection with them so we can finally hear their deeper message and understand their purpose. It feels uncomfortable and horrible to think that these thoughts are the real us. But we have been carrying these thoughts and feelings for thousands of years. They are just showing up in you because your ancestors used the same approach to life. Future generations have an opportunity to co-create a very different reality. To give them this opportunity, you just have to heal from an addiction you didn't know you had.

It was an uncomfortable moment for a client of mine when he realized he had been lying to himself for years, telling himself he wasn't an angry person. But one day, when he couldn't handle his child anymore, he lashed out, assuring me he didn't recognize this person. "That isn't me," he repeated. The harsh reality was very different. He had just used his military training to control his honest thoughts and feelings. That is until the raging bull escaped after being cooped up for so long to reveal how he had honestly felt all his life.

As a consequence of this ancient and stoic approach to life, we've become so good at denial we don't realize just how often we are lying to ourselves. It postpones us from realizing it isn't what we do, view, or listen to that ultimately impacts us. We are unconsciously seeking out certain social media posts, movies, and podcasts to help us discover our honest state of mind. We don't randomly choose what to watch on the latest streaming service. Our decisions and choices originate from whatever is in our foundation. When you are feeling victimized and angry, your choice of what you watch and eat will be different from when you feel motivated and have meaning.

How can we be happy when we are constantly on alert, believing we could be held back, tricked, and hijacked at any point by the very thing we take everywhere with us? And then told the answer is to get better at lying to ourselves?

Bored of victimizing myself and bullying the so-called bullies in my life, I started to seek out any place I gave myself wiggle room to get my blame fix. No rock was left unturned. Which was helpful because I found it hiding just about everywhere I looked.

Bullying the Bully

Have you ever started a fight with your girlfriend the night before a big social event? Or called your dad to talk about Christmas plans, only to have the conversation turn into an argument about why you can't get a better job? Or had brunch with your sister, only to get into a yelling match about why she maliciously tried to flush your toy penguin down the toilet when you were four?

Sometimes we enlist others to distribute blame so we can get what we want while continuing to play the Blame Game. Maybe we want to leave a relationship, gain our parent's

117

approval, or convince our sister to help us out financially. So we start a fight with our partner, call our dad an overcritical ass, or tell our sister she's selfish and unsupportive. These strategies can be effective in helping us get what we truly want, but what are the side effects?

Take bullying, for example. I know firsthand that being picked on is a horrible, painful, and humiliating experience. And when it was happening, I considered myself the innocent victim. But in retrospect, I realized it wasn't as one-sided as I thought. The label "bully" is given to someone who is looking to harm someone they see as vulnerable. In a society where blame addiction is rampant and we are being encouraged to be more vulnerable—which means to be open to attack or being harmed—it is no wonder this victim/bully relationship is so prevalent. For this dynamic to change, our approach needs to dramatically alter. We have to move from victimizing the victim and bullying the bully to realizing it is a relationship we co-create to help us with important feedback.

Between the ages of five and eighteen, I collected a number of bullies. I despised my teenage bully. I was always anticipating him and waiting for him to jump out of nowhere like a lion pouncing on its innocent prey. I hid my troubles from my parents as best I could, until my schoolwork showed signs that all was not well. I mostly closed down, but sometimes my honesty erupted into violent outbursts of frustration. When my parents did find out what was happening at school, I received sympathy from my mother and the advice to "hit the biggest guy first" from my father.

Despite my protests, eventually my mother got the school involved. But before the school could do anything, everything changed—well, with this particular bully. I was walking to my English class, consumed with the fear of being asked to read out loud at the front of the room. My bully came out of nowhere and pushed me so hard that I flew backwards and fell on the floor. Instead of my usual timid victim response to this, I jumped up and aggressively shouted and confronted my bully in what could only have been a terrifying scene for him and everyone else watching. I was so stressed by other things going on in my personal life like my parents' separation and upcoming exams that I had "forgotten" to play my role as victim.

The confrontation with my childhood bully led me to take up weight training and martial arts in case something similar happened again. Interestingly enough, they became lifelong pursuits. The confidence that my fighting skills brought turned to bravado. However, the hardened exterior was only a facade, and it covered up the gaping hole where my self-esteem could have been. I didn't heal from my blame addiction when I confronted my bully that day. I enjoyed the reprieve, but it wasn't long before the next one stepped in to show me that I was still in the Victim Cycle.

It took years to realize that my bullies were my teachers. It might not have been their conscious or altruistic goal, but that doesn't negate the point that they were doing all they could to show me I was being a victim. We don't see this because we keep feeding our addiction and blaming them.

When does motivation become bullying? At what point does a supportive and encouraging parent become annoying and interfering? How many bullies must we endure before we realize maybe we need to heal and become honestly confident rather than place our focus on them changing or how to avoid them? How many evenings must we agree to work late before we stop thinking our boss is taking advantage of us and start realizing we have contributed to this dynamic? How many "crazy" exes do we need to cycle through before we admit we are the common denominator? Is there a possibility that we might be unknowingly choosing these people specifically and unconsciously orchestrating these breakups because we don't actually know ourselves?

A client once came to me complaining that her husband was bullying her and always accused her of being a victim. A few minutes into her tirade, I stopped my client and confirmed her husband's accusations. "You do realize every one of your stories places you as the innocent victim," I said. They all reinforced the belief that her husband and others were the problem, and she was simply the innocent bystander. Thinking I was defending her husband, she defended her stance, not recognizing how ingrained her victimhood had become in her psyche.

After years of perfecting and orating her victim stories to friends and family, her mind was closed to any possibility that she contributed in any way to what occurred in her life, especially when it came to her husband. As the session went on, she regularly interrupted me to say, "You tell me, is this the act of a nice and kind man…" and then proceeded to tell me all the bad, negative, and wrong things he did and all the good, positive, and right things she did. When I offered alternative viewpoints, she would give me more "evidence" to confirm her mantra, "I do everything right and I always get punished for it!"

I asked my client, "What do you think is the reason some people get bullied and others don't?" She focused on people's appearance. I suggested it was more to do with someone's energy (inner confidence). A bully will scan a classroom, playground, office, or boardroom and pick up on body language as well as the energy emanating from everyone. When they perceive a vulnerability, they go over and test the market to see if they will agree to engage in the victim/bully relationship.

I asked her, "Who do you think needs to change for your relationship with your husband to change?"

"Him!" was her immediate and well-practiced response.

My client was of Chinese descent, so I asked, "If I told you I can't wait for 1.4 billion people to change for me to be happy, I am sure you would see the issue with my happiness plan." She nodded in agreement. When the numbers are reduced to one or two people, however, we lose sight of this wisdom and think it is *them* that need to change, not *us*. But of course this is how a victim sees life.

People in this mindset hand out labels like candy on Halloween. It is easy to go from healthy friend to toxic if you do something they deem as unsupportive. After years of going from obese to showing off your hard work on Instagram, you go from inspirational to narcissistic. Labeling people like this is one-dimensional thinking and it keeps us in the Blame Game. Conflict and dissatisfaction only exist when blame is in the air. When we jump to a blame-based conclusion, we delay the opportunity to honestly self-reflect. To realize the very accusations we are throwing around might actually be directed at ourselves. It isn't always a comfortable moment when we realize that we might have the same "narcissistic" tendencies as the person we are pointing at.

The victim/bully relationship is actually a victim/victim one. They are both showing their insecurities in different ways and become magnetized to each other. I say this not to prove we are in a Marvel movie but so we can all honestly heal and experience the freedom that comes with being honestly confident where sexual, physical, and psychological abusive behavior no longer exists in our lives.

We have more to contribute to our lives than we might realize. We just have to think like a freak, as the Freakonomics guys would say, and think differently while taking an uncomfortable dive into our self-honesty to see how.

We Are All Contributing

When couples come into my sessions, they often arrive fully loaded with blame and ready for a shoot-out at sundown. Familiar comments include, "Bob stays at the office late every night. I know he could get home for dinner if he really wanted to. He's so selfish and only thinks of himself!" and "I don't know what I did wrong to make Bob not want to spend time with me!"

Not to worry—Bob has a lot of blame bombs in his arsenal as well. "I don't know why Carol just can't understand that I'm working to provide for our family. She's so ungrateful." Sometimes when the air is thick with blame, I use a provocative strategy and turn to one of them first.

"You do realize," I say to Bob, "that you created this."

Usually Carol smiles and crosses her arms in satisfaction, happy to receive validation that she is right; the whole situation is all Bob's fault. I then turn to Carol and tell her exactly the same thing. I advise both of them that they are wholly responsible for the situation. They are participating in co-creation. It takes two to create any interpersonal dynamic. For deep and honest healing to take place, both partners will need to take 100 percent blame-free responsibility for their contribution.

This is not another way of saying it is our "fault." Any focus on blaming ourselves or the other person keeps us in the Victim Cycle and disrupts the perfectly designed self-reflection and self-honesty process.

Co-creation means that each one of us is contributing to every experience we have. This idea can come off as incredibly offensive if we are in the midst of a painful situation or doing all we can to block out a past traumatic event. It might sound like I'm negating someone's lived experience, or "victim blaming," but of course this is not the case. Realizing you are a creator and taking blame-free responsibility for your part in the co-creation is not about blaming in any shape or form. Rather it's about recognizing that all parties involved have known and unknown motivations that are constantly playing out. The underlying one is that we are bringing to life an unknown addiction that has been thousands of years in the making. An addiction that leads us to think life is unfair and full of evil. And the acceptance of this narrative brings it to reality.

The reason why this premise can cause such defensive reactions is because we have become so reliant on self-control that we have numbed ourselves to our self-honesty. It doesn't look nice to others if we share our fantasy of getting revenge on an ex or share the fact that we still maintain a grudge against our parents. In a similar way, we don't like to think we remain single so we don't get hurt, avoid speaking in public to protect us from humiliation, or any number of things. We might have glimpses now and then that we have these honest feelings. But because we think they are not healthy or that acting on them would ostracize us from friends and family, we remain in the Victim Cycle.

It was incredibly challenging for me to entertain the idea I was co-creating events that I had spent a lifetime believing I had no contribution to—I was the innocent victim. It was only after starting to discover blame's influence in my life and hearing thousands of stories from clients that I came up with a hypothesis: that we are constantly co-creating ever more extreme situations to help us with our overriding goal—to break through our thick layers of control, acceptance, and denial so we can finally get to know who we honestly are.

My client Alex made remarkable progress understanding himself through recognizing his deep self-honesty and his role as a co-creator. His wife, Rebecca, had resigned from her job without discussing it with him. Rebecca had not secured another position before quitting and had no contingency plan. Alex blamed Rebecca for jeopardizing their financial security and considered himself an innocent victim.

To help Alex wrap his mind around the idea that he con-tributed to his current situation, I asked him to think about any areas of his home and work life that were different since Rebecca suddenly left her job. I wanted him to entertain the possibility that he had contributed to and actually benefited from his wife's decision in some way. I pushed him out of his comfort zone (denial) in order to lift the rug, open the door, and unscrew the lid to give him access to his self-honesty.

"The only thing I can think of," Alex responded, "is that I am happy she is happier." He then shared how his wife was like a different person after quitting her job. She had been miserable for months, and it was a relief to have Rebecca back to her usual self. I asked him if this had impacted his work at all. At that moment, he sat back in his chair and recalled how since her seemingly irrational decision, his relationship with his boss had mysteriously improved and he had closed more deals. Of course, this could have been a coincidence if you believe in such things, but he admitted that he didn't realize just how much his wife's unhappiness over the previous six months had impacted him. When he was at work, a lot of his attention (worry) was with his wife.

Even though he could now see the benefits, Alex admitted there was still part of him that thought what his wife did was wrong. He felt she should have done the "right" thing and consulted him before making such a drastic decision. He felt a little more comfortable taking *partial* responsibility, but not *full* blame-free responsibility, for his part. He was still playing the Blame Game, which kept him feeling like a victim. His attachment to his wife doing the wrong thing came from his denial that he had more to contribute. He was effectively lying to himself without knowing it. I pushed him to think about how his own actions might have led his wife to make this move. It was a light-bulb moment for him when he remembered how he actually encouraged her to leave her job on a number of occasions. Then it dawned on him that, unbeknownst to him until our session, Rebecca's happiness was higher on his priority list than he realized. Thus, he was finally able to take full blame-free responsibility for his part in co-creating her resignation.

Like many of my clients, Alex was resistant when I first told him that he would benefit from taking 100 percent blame-free responsibility for his role in co-creating Rebecca's sudden unemployment. Like many of the people I offer self-honesty and co-creation to, he initially thought I was rehashing the *take radical responsibility for your life* advice, where he should bear all the fault on his shoulders. Alex was initially frustrated because he believed I was justifying his wife's behavior. On the contrary, I wasn't releasing his wife from responsibility at all. I wanted her to take 100 percent blame-free responsibility too. My goal wasn't to transfer blame from one person to another but to show Alex (and his wife) what honest freedom and liberation feels like and what it results in.

It was fascinating to see that as soon as they both exited their victimhood, Rebecca, after months of not being able to find a new position, effortlessly secured her ideal job with more money and responsibility. And for Alex, with his wife's happiness clinched and financial stability assured, he noticed how he effortlessly made decisions to optimize his health, which he had wanted to do for years. When his foundation changed, his decisions naturally changed. There was no conscious choice involved. He consciously executed what had already been unconsciously decided.

The challenge we face is to take responsibility for our contribution while sensing whether we are transferring the blame onto ourselves. Seeing things as "all our fault" or viewing ourselves as being "our own worst enemy" casts us as victims of our own actions. This puts us into a state of fear, uncertainty, and doubt. And while in this state, the last place we want to venture into is the part of us we have dedicated a lifetime to controlling and pushing away because we are convinced it is holding us back—our self-honesty.

CHAPTER 8

The Strongest Force in Nature

When we ignore the whispers of self-honesty, the whispering becomes talking, which becomes shouting, which eventually becomes screaming, until we finally *listen* (or not). This process is akin to trash building up on a beach. When there is only one plastic bag in the sand, no one cares much. But as more garbage piles up, people notice and organize community cleanups, install trash cans, and institute steep fines for littering. When the beach fills up with rubbish, it becomes more work to achieve the goal.

Similarly, it's far less work to heal when we listen to the signs *earlier*. And even less effort is needed when we are in the prevention rather than the cure mindset. We innately know this, but the Blame Game has us covering our eyes until we trip over an old tire and finally decide the beach needs cleaning.

Mark came to me saying he was done with high-maintenance women who always create drama in his life and instead wanted to find a cool and collected woman. To him, it appeared that anytime he walked into a room, the most dramatic woman would zero in on him, and he would feel magnetically drawn to her. The relationship would never work and eventually go down in flames, just like all his previous ones. He'd spin into a blame cycle, blasting women in general and himself. In our workshops, he repeatedly used the words "always" and "never," a testament to his narrowed blame-addicted mindset.

Many times, when we are deep in the Blame Game like Mark, we forget we are often pulled toward the people who reflect back our self-honesty. The escalating patterns might feel like things are getting worse, but maybe they provide us with opportunities to gain new awareness about ourselves. It is often easier to see in others what needs to change for them to heal and experience a different life. That's why it is helpful to see others as a mirror who reflect back the parts in ourselves that we can't see need addressing.

For Mark, his blame addiction was strong. He reveled in victimhood. He needed ever-increasing amounts of sympathy and drama to sustain himself. He liked to have the *worst* victim experience in the room. He could frequently be heard chiming in, "You think that's bad? Well, let me tell you what happened to me!" On one level, this meant he could continue to blame and punish his parents for his perceived less-than-ideal upbringing and their drawn-out emotionally taxing divorce that supposedly messed him up when he was a young child. Ultimately, he didn't realize he kept co-creating difficult relationships, not because he was repeating self-sabotaging patterns, but to give himself opportunities to get honest with himself and heal from his blame addiction.

During our first session, I stopped Mark in his tracks and said, "I am stopping you like I do with many of my clients when they are feeding their 'poor me' stories." It sounded harsh, but I wanted to disrupt the dynamic he was used to with his friends, family, and therapists. By constantly listening to the same one-dimensional version of his reality, everyone was feeding his unknown addiction. My comment was designed to shake him into realizing that the way he perceived his stories was keeping him in the Victim Cycle, and his mind, body, and surroundings were screaming at him for relief. And when I shook his Poor Me tree, down came all the Poor Me leaves, leaving Mark with just the self-honest roots and bare branches of possibilities to explore.

This was a shock to his system. Mark felt confused as the shimmering mirage faded away and revealed his self-honesty. He felt held back by women and was very comfortable blaming women for all his dating problems. Earlier in our sessions he told me he felt no blame toward his mother and that we should focus on other people in his life. He used to "hate" her, but now they have a great relationship. It was only when the bare branches were exposed that he broke down and confessed his honest feelings and that he had used untold amounts of self-control to keep the relationship going.

There is no force stronger than our self-honesty. Regardless of what we put in its way, it will continue to push through so it can be heard. We will keep co-creating ever more extreme experiences to help us break through our denial, ignorance, or any techniques we have implemented to reprogram, rewire, or reset our thoughts and beliefs.

Take my client Joan as an example. For many years, she had been searching for a loving partner and over that time had amassed a laundry list of complaints about what was wrong with men and with herself. She had found the label "abandonment issues" on the internet and found it helpful for explaining the aftereffects of her father leaving her as a child. After all the self-work she had done, she still couldn't understand why she attracted men who she described as emotionally unavailable.

Joan came to me very frustrated, lamenting that something was blocking her, and according to a blog she read, it was her self-sabotaging thoughts that were holding her back from finding a faithful long-term companion. As an avid advocate of the law of attraction, Joan was adept with the tools she had learned to help her get what she consciously wanted. She hoped that based on the latest research around neuroplasticity, she could train her brain with intense visualization to create new neural pathways that would manifest her soulmate. She also proudly told me she had read *The Power of Now* by Eckhart Tolle and had learnt to just accept her current situation to gain power over it, think positive thoughts to attract positivity, and let go of her negative past. All so she can be in the moment where the worries of the past and the future become irrelevant.

Joan didn't know this exact approach was full of blame, which is why she remained in the Victim Cycle regardless of how many times she read the book, meditated, or visualized her soulmate. She was learning how to become even more dishonest with herself. To help her access her deeper honesty, I let her know that I like to keep life very simple. I used to overcomplicate every situation by all the philosophies and techniques I had accumulated. I offered that I now look at the facts I am presented with—the facts that are indisputable, not my version of them.

I said, "Up to this very moment I know you don't whole-heartedly want a long-term loving relationship." "How can you say such a thing?" she shot back. After many relationships and dates, it looked like she 100 percent wanted to find a partner. There was evidence for all to see. But again, when we are no longer in blame or acceptance, much more can rise to the top.

How could I be so confident? Simply because the undisputed fact remained, Joan had never had a long-term loving relationship and wasn't in one at the time of our session. I know part of her wanted to be in one, but the majority (even if that was 51 percent) didn't. I followed this up with the suggestion that we needed to address the part of her that didn't want it rather than keep pushing the lie that 100 percent of her did want a long-term partner.

Initially, she balked at the suggestion. It was too simple and counterintuitive to her other teachings. She assured me she DID want a loving partner. It was her negative thoughts and patterns that were blocking her. She had been taught to focus on her con-scious desire of finding her twin flame. Any other way of thinking would be considered negative and bring about more negativity. She had a vision board and religiously recited her morning posi-tive mantras and finished the day with her gratitude diary. All in the hope the "universe" or her "higher-self" would deliver what she told them to bring. I know these ideas and techniques can bring amazing short-term results. They helped me tremendously when I knew no better. But it is an exhausting way to live, and as soon as our energy runs out, which it had for Joan, self-honesty shoots through and no amount of self-control or gratitude journaling will work to stop it.

I asked Joan, "How is being single helping you right now?"

"It's not!" she blasted back.

Entrenched in her victimhood, she continued to blame her father for her abandonment issues and herself for her health conditions that drove away dating prospects. I took Joan through a process to give her access to her self-honesty. Part of that process was to repeat the question in a different way: "What are possible reasons you might want to be single or not want to be in a long-term relationship?" We went back and forth a few times until we broke through her denial. When she finally spoke, she said, "If I am going to be honest Denis, my priority has been to build a career and be financially secure." She admitted that being single had allowed her to devote time to finishing an important project two years in the making. She wasn't ready to give her time and freedom to someone else. This helped explain why she wasn't in a relationship now, but she still struggled with the idea that she didn't wholeheartedly want one in the past.

It is tempting to jump down a rabbit hole and find out all the reasons that could make Joan choose this route in life. Why does she think relationships are time consuming and constraining? What happened in her previous relationships to make her feel this way? What was her relationship like with her mother? But this line of digging would be coming from a place that considered her choices bad or wrong, based on what society has deemed ideal for her gender, age, religion, or cultural position.

Through listening to herself honestly, she discovered all the perceived setbacks and mistakes had actually led her to achieve her honest desire. She had an independent streak running through her veins since birth. She liked to travel and have as many adventures as she could. It was a different story for her sister. She wanted to find a husband and settle down in one place and have a family. And that is what she effortlessly co-created. They were brought up under the same house, but they both had very different honest desires. Joan was trying to replicate her sister's perceived success to please her parents, but it didn't match what she genuinely wanted.

This realization opened her up to the possibility she had more input in what happens in her life than she thought. She had been dishonest with herself and every man she met. When they got serious and talked about settling down in one place, she felt uncomfortable because she needed to feel free and independent. She had to experience what life had to offer and she had the means to do that. However, she always stuck to the line she was looking for marriage and children, which she wasn't. She needed variety whereas her sister needed stability.

Self-honesty is an important ingredient that makes up the antidote to our blame addiction and enables us to exit the Victim Cycle. Blaming herself became a little harder because she acknowledged how her past situation was actually in line with her honest priorities. It was also more difficult to blame men for being unavailable because she realized she was actually also being unavailable.

In the weeks that followed, Joan mentioned she felt calmer and noticed changes in her life. She felt more ready (and honest) to find a loving partner, but mentioned she still hadn't found "the one." After helping her realize this search was full of attachment (blame) and *the one* is whoever she is with at that time, she met someone who she described as "not the type of person I would normally be attracted to." I never found out how long this relationship lasted, but she had been single for three years and the fact she met someone the day after this session was a reflection of how much she had healed from her blame addiction.

We are always co-creating every situation to give us a reality check. I have said in the past that "life is a bullshit meter." It is relentlessly showing us whether we are being honest with ourselves or not. Because we are all so individual, we all have different ideals around what constitutes an extreme experience. To simplify the recovery process, the goal is to focus on the feelings and where they show up in our body, not the actual details of the events. Getting caught in the weeds of "he did this, she did that," might feel justifiable, but it always leads to more repressed anger and conflict. It is exhausting.

The best bullshit meter we have is our body. It is always letting us know if we are being honest with ourselves or not.

Mind-Body Connection

Looking down at her feet, one of my workshop participants exclaimed, "My toes are bending! My toes are bending!" For this nineteen-year-old dancer, it was a life-changing moment. She had been diagnosed with juvenile arthritis at the age of thirteen and, for the past six years, could not move the toes on her left foot, not even so much as a wiggle.

Moments earlier I explained to the participants how our body is always helping us and nudging us toward self-honesty.

The dancer recalled what was happening in her life just before she was diagnosed with juvenile arthritis at age thirteen. She had wanted to quit ballet, but she kept her feelings to herself because she was too scared to let her parents and teachers down. They loved her dancing and had invested significant time, energy, and resources to get her to a high standard. In our workshop she had a moment of deep honesty. She realized how her label of juvenile arthritis was her unconscious way of getting what she deeply wanted but felt she couldn't consciously pursue. When she lost the ability to move her toes, she suddenly had a guilt-free reason to stop ballet. Now her parents could be disappointed with the label of arthritis and not with their *daughter*.

When we remove the label, we are just left with the fact that her body was talking to her. It helped her get what she honestly wanted six years ago. In theory, she didn't need to go down this road, but everyone in her ecosystem (family) were unknowingly in the Victim Cycle. This meant playing the victim helped her out of a difficult situation, like it helped me when I got my sister to stop picking on me by biting my arm. The difference was, I very aware of what I was doing, and she wasn't. She unconsciously achieved her honest goal by playing the Blame Game. But this also kept her in a state of dishonesty, which her toes were constantly reminding her of. Once she accessed that self-honesty, her toes were free from their purpose—to show her she was playing the Blame Game and being dishonest.

I used to believe the mind-body connection was tenuous at best, but after witnessing "arthritis" disappear, "frozen shoulders" become mobile, and "autoimmune" disorders reverse within a matter of weeks, hours, and sometimes minutes, I can tell you with confidence that profound physical change is possible. More than that, it's not miraculous at all. In fact, it's quite normal once you understand that our mental and physical health is seamlessly connected to self-honesty.

The lady with the now bendy toes was shocked at what happened. She had accepted the doctors' diagnosis that she would have to learn to live with arthritis for the rest of her life. In order to help everyone grasp what happened, I asked the group, "Have you ever made plans with friends, and as the date gets closer, you start to dread the energy and effort it will take to go out? And then the day before you mysteriously come down with a cold?" The room filled with reluctant nods. I posed a second question: "Even though you might or might not have been sick on those occasions, did you immediately feel better after you sent the message to cancel?" Chuckles escaped from the participants. This is a common phenomenon many people can relate to.

When we do this, we get what we want without being honest. We are often too afraid of being blamed for being a "bad friend" so we lie, even if we justify that it is only a little one. It is like using your children to escape a boring dinner party or a sick pet for why you can't commit to a fundraising event. It seems harmless. And at the beginning, we could argue that it is. But the longer we use this strategy, we don't realize how lying to ourselves and others becomes our normal. Soon we are making up ailments, car problems, family members visiting from overseas, and unexpected bug infestations for why we can't do things. But at what point is it enough? Is it when we find ourselves hiding behind the couch when there is a knock at the door or bribing our kids to play along?

The longer it goes on, the longer we remain ignorant that we are co-creators. We deny our friend the opportunity to show us that they didn't want to go out either but was also doing the right thing. We teach each other how to become expert liars without realizing it because we are expert blamers.

Mirror, Mirror on the Wall

The other interesting piece of co-creation is that we often un-knowingly recruit other people to mirror our emotions and insecurities back to us so we can get more honest with ourselves. We might like to think opposites attract, but I've found birds of a feather flock together as well. The complexity of human behav-ior can be perplexing. But as I have mentioned, it can be simple when we gain more awareness around our blame addiction. We will draw people in so we can serve as mirrors of each other.

"My mother was terrible and she ruined my life!" Jane, a mother of two, told me in her first session.

I hear this type of complaint often. Jane had recently been in a big argument with her husband, which escalated after he said, "You are just like your mother." She said she hated hear-ing that because she was doing all she could to not be like her mom. She didn't want to bring her kids up in the same awful way she was raised. Her defensive walls were up, her blinkers were on, and her blame finger was poised on the trigger ready to rattle off a list of examples showcasing how her mother and husband were the cause of her misery.

"Okay, let's do a creative exercise," I said. I asked her to get a plain piece of paper and at the top of the page write the name of the person or persons she was most angry with. In order to facilitate accessing the most self-honesty, I assured her that whatever she wrote was for her eyes only. I said, "It is like when a doctor asks you how much alcohol you drink or how many cigarettes you smoke. We want to tell the truth, but a lie reflex kicks in and we smudge the truth a little." We do this because we don't want to be seen as a bad person. Knowing that she could tell me anything she wanted—or not reveal anything and destroy the list after the exercise—put her at ease. With that said, she told me she wrote down her mother and husband.

"Great," I said. "Now when I give you the next instruction, I want you to write down the answer as a stream of consciousness, again in the knowledge that whatever you write is ultimately for you, not me. The goal is to write bullet points of whatever comes to mind without pause."

Under both of the names I asked her to write down all the things she didn't like about them. All the characteristics, traits, and behaviors that made her annoyed, disappointed, sad, frustrated, or angry. After a few minutes she told me there were eleven points she could think of. To which I said, "How would you feel if you just wrote a list about yourself?" "Not too happy," she said.

As a way of explaining the next part of the exercise, I shared another client example. I received an emergency call from David. His back had locked up and he could barely move without excruciating pain. He was frustrated and angry. I asked him, "Who did you recently have an argument with?" His immediate response was denial. I understood why he was reluctant to share. He had been clinically diagnosed with "anger issues" and didn't want to come across as not doing a good job controlling his outbursts. I suggested that his tense and *inflamed* back was telling us he was very much feeding his blame addiction, and I assumed it was because of something someone did. After a brief pause, he blurted out, "If I am going to be honest, it is my brother. He is so stubborn. He never listens to me."

I explained to Jane that David was actually angry and frustrated with his own stubbornness, which was being reflected back to him by his brother. He didn't like that he had the same trait, as it often caused stress in his marriage. His wife often accused him of not listening to her, which was another complaint he had about his brother. I asked Jane to look over her eleven bullet points and mark any of them that she could own as a direct reflection of her own character or behavior, making sure she thought about all relationships and aspects of her life not just in relation to her mother and husband. She told me that there were eight she recognized. It felt uncomfortable to admit, she told me, but if she was being honest, she behaved in a similar way sometimes with different people in her life.

Blaming others for our unhappiness holds up a mirror to ourselves. We haven't been encouraged to take notice of the small mirrors, the slight twinkle of a reflection showing us early on what needs our attention. If we did, then we could address the experience when it wouldn't be classed as bad, negative, or wrong, and the task would be painless and effortless. The reality is: Jane blamed her mother for a poor upbringing and was terrified to repeat the pattern with her own children. Her husband had become her replacement punching bag because he was bringing their children up in the same (wrong) way.

The "mirror exercise" has one main goal: to recognize that the person you are blaming isn't the enemy. Unknowingly, they are helping you by reflecting back the self-honesty you have spent a lifetime hiding from. It is a little bit harder to blame others when you are open to the possibility that they are helping you (albeit unconsciously) rather than holding you back.

This isn't always the most comfortable of exercises at the start, because it replaces the "control" part of the Victim Cycle and disrupts the rotation. But as I explained to Jane, it is like starting a new high-intensity interval training (HIIT) workout program. It isn't always comfortable at first, but you get to a point where you look forward to sweating and pushing yourself out of your comfort zone. The mirror exercise is the HIIT of mental and emotional healing.

This was a big revelation for Jane. It was a shock to admit that, while she was accusing her mother of "being negative and controlling all the time," her husband was frequently directing the same criticism at her. Jane admitted she was often quick to criticize her husband and kids for not doing what she wanted them to do. Upon reflection, she could see how militant she often was toward homework and certain tasks around the house. She ran quite a dictatorship.

There were a few things she wrote on the list that didn't resonate with her at all. I assured her this is normal. There are things that we really don't want to come face-to-face with. It is like having two mirrors in your home. One has the uncanny ability to make you look fat, old, and tired; the other has great lighting that brings out the features you like. Which mirror would you want to avoid?

She told me that her mother was physically "violent." Jane was quick to assure me that she has never been violent.

"So you have never thought about hitting your children?" I asked her.

"Well, of course it may have crossed my mind, but I've never acted on it," she replied.

I pushed further and asked, "Have you ever gotten angry with another person when driving, or have you ever wanted to hit or throw something at your husband?" After a little hesitation, she confidently said she'd never had road rage, but there had been many times when violent thoughts entered her mind regarding her husband. This had happened more recently, as they were going through a difficult time in their marriage. She again assured me she had never acted on any of the thoughts and recently took up jogging to help if they became too much to handle.

Basically, she had learned to control that part of herself. It was extremely uncomfortable to recognize all the remaining bullet points on her page were a reflection of what she was doing or had used control to stop herself from doing. Self-control is merely a facade. It is not a magical shield that is impervious to our self-honesty. It has to come out at some point. Jane also wrote down "selfish" and again assured me that she was always thinking of others. So I asked if she thought being selfish was bad. "Of course!" she said. I asked how she would feel if I said, "The most important person in the world is you."

In a world where we throw around labels like "narcissist" and "egotistical" like greetings, it feels normal to put others before ourselves. It can get quite confusing when we are being told to love ourselves one minute and not to think too much of ourselves the next. Joan felt incredibly uncomfortable to think of herself in that way. That was until she exited the Victim Cycle and found a new sense of confidence she hadn't experienced before. And what's more, the more she looked after herself, the more connected she felt to everyone else and the more she wanted to help others.

The mirror exercise is designed to give us access to all sides of ourselves. It illustrates that every time we blame others, we are effectively shooting the messenger because they are simply reflecting back the parts of us that we deem ugly and wrong.

I mentioned to Jane that she could do the reverse of this exercise and write down all the things she liked about her mother and husband (or anyone for that matter). That would help her see the parts she liked most about herself. This can create equally uncomfortable feelings as we also don't acknowledge these attributes. But if they are in others, they are in us. We are drawn to others who reflect back what we want and need to see. We are constantly co-creating situations with our loved ones, as they have the uncanny ability to hit the nerves that we thought we had protected the most.

The driving force behind what we co-create in our lives is not the fake positive one we offer the world. Life can feel like a constant battle because our self-honesty is relentless at pushing through any wall we put up to show us that this is where we ultimately co-create our reality.

All It Takes Is One Piece of Information

All the while we are in the Blame Game where control is a key factor, we have a fragile existence where every interaction can leave us either feeling like an empowered and joyful go-getter or a helpless victim. It is a fine line we constantly walk.

But what if you are actually co-creating all the situations in your life to help you get to a place of deeper self-honesty so you can heal and finally get to know the real you?

For example, imagine that after running from the taxi to the check-in counter at the airport, you find out you missed your flight. Most people would be furious, especially if they could blame something obvious like the taxi driver, unexpected traffic, or the meeting that went way overtime. But what happens if you find out that the plane you were supposed to be on crashed? You might experience a sense of relief. You may suddenly feel gratitude for the taxi driver, traffic, or lengthy meeting. In one nanosecond you went from wanting to hit the taxi driver to wanting to hug him for saving your life. With one piece of information, you went from blaming life, God, or the universe for not having your back to being amazed at how magical life is and how lucky you are.

Situations we perceive as bad or unhelpful feel totally out of our control, so we perceive them as negative because they seem to be ruining our plans. This is especially true if there is no obvious benefit. If there isn't a taxi driver to blame, we might point the finger at our friend who spent too long getting coffee on the way to the airport, whoever designed the overpass and made it totally confusing, or the airline because they did a horrible job coordinating flights during a thunderstorm. Or we might blame ourselves. We should have left the hotel earlier, read the signs more carefully, and planned more time between flights. The pattern is so familiar: this sucks, so whose fault is it?

But what if we had more of a contribution to these types of experiences than we first think? I encourage clients to once again train their perception muscle. I ask them to come up with as many possible reasons as to why someone might honestly want to have their conscious travel plans foiled. Maybe they were on the way to give a talk they weren't prepared for. Or they might have been on the way to a beach vacation where their friends would see their embarrassing bikini rash. Or they didn't want to go on a romantic getaway with their partner because they were having an affair. Spending time with a sick parent or a new kitten at home could be more of a priority than a weekend hiking in the rain. When I redirect them to look at their own blame-based stories, they realize they achieved their honest desire, just not in the way they consciously wanted.

A client who I took through this very scenario told me how it happened to him. He was furious with the taxi driver for making him and his boss miss a flight. And because the plane landed safely, he remained a victim of circumstance. It took a while of jousting, but after he got self-honest, he admitted he was dreading the trip. He had a phobia of public speaking, and he was going to present to a thousand people in front of his new boss. He finally admitted he knew the driver was going the long way but didn't say anything, wishing they would miss the flight. Like the lady in the juvenile arthritis example, he was invested in believing his own story because other people had to buy into the victim story. His boss was in the car with him. He had to match his boss's sense of hardship so he didn't get found out.

For honest healing to take place, we must realize that on some level we don't wholeheartedly want something to happen if it didn't happen. At the start of the honest healing process, it requires an uncomfortable level of self-honesty and self-reflection to become aware of our contribution to what happens in our lives. We have been taught to focus on the perceived positive, so we stick to the story that we absolutely, unequivocally wanted our conscious plan to happen. There is a genuine fear, that if they explore the possible reasons, which they consider negative, that they will somehow manifest more negative outcomes. This whole approach to life falls apart when we start to delve into our self-honesty, and remember just how subjective, relative, and multidimensional each experience is.

Many of my clients tell me victim-based stories where people have lied to them. Sometimes it is a little annoying lie, while other times it is a story about being betrayed. It can be an uncomfortable feeling when I show them just how much they lie to themselves and others. So what do you think others will mirror back to you if you are lying to yourself all the time?

For example, a client told me they were angry with their partner for cheating on them after seven years of marriage. After some back and forth, they reluctantly answered my question, "When did you honestly want to leave the relationship?" Finally being honest, they said, "After about five years things changed. I tried so hard to get it back to what it was, but we just argued more and more. It became unbearable." Because they saw divorce as failure, they were prepared to stick it out through whatever happened. But they were getting more mentally and physically ill to a point they couldn't ignore what they really wanted. Ultimately, even though it looked like one side made the decision, it was both of them. It had to be so extreme because they wouldn't have made the decision otherwise. For honest healing to take place, we benefit from focusing on *our* contribution and not *theirs*.

The honest healing process is paradoxical, as it is a selfish journey but has a selfless outcome. When you honestly heal and exit the Victim Cycle, your ecosystem has to adapt and heal also. Everyone has different personality traits that they show different people. It is why someone can be described as "horrible" by one person and "kind" by another. When you honestly heal, the people in your life will reflect your own changes back to you.

CHAPTER 9

The Habit of Self-Blame

Self-blame is at the heart of our blame addiction. It is constantly there in the back of our minds, shuffling through victim stories like a maxed-out iPod on repeat. With our trained self-discipline, we play around with the volume, doing all we can to distract or numb ourselves in the hope of finally letting them go. However, our control-based strategies have the effect of putting a plant in front of a cracked tile in the kitchen and thinking the problem is solved. Out of sight out of mind. But the same thoughts and stories are always there taking up mental real estate, requiring an ever-depleting amount of energy to keep up the hope that the plant will magically fix the cracked tile.

There is a reason why we constantly seek our blame fix by pointing the finger straight back at ourselves. We relentlessly accept the notion that we are self-sabotaging and holding ourselves back. This is drummed into us from a young age, and our acceptance of it makes self-blame a loyal companion.

New clients come to me fully loaded with self-blame rhetoric they have picked up on their self-development journey: "I am hindering my own success," "I think maybe *I'm* the toxic one," or "I keep sabotaging all my relationships." It makes sense because we are constantly told we are standing in our own way. It is our harmful, destructive, and negative thoughts, patterns, and behaviors that are blocking us from reaching our dreams. It leads to that repetitive line of questioning, "Why me? Why do I keep doing this to myself? Why is life so unfair?"

These teachings are front and center whether the client is aware of it or not. It is why they can get very defensive when I introduce them to the idea that we have more to contribute to our painful experiences than we realize. Their rebuttals can sound something like, "You are saying I wanted and created my best friend betraying me! Why would I create such horrible people and events in my life?" It can sound implausible that we have something to contribute to these events, but that is only because we have evolved into a species that relies on control as a means of functioning and predominantly thinks in black and white. After thousands of years hearing the relentless echoing of the same blame-based advice and philosophy, our minds resemble a closed walnut. And like a walnut might need some strong coaxing or a swift hit to open up, this is what the rest of the book is about.

We have been encouraged by unknown blame addicts to follow their advice. It has resulted in us spending a lifetime blaming, lying, and beating ourselves up. Is it any wonder why others would do the same back to us? Are we not fulfilling the

Golden Rule? Do not do to others what you would not like done to yourself. On the surface it sounds like a great ethos for life. Consciously we want to be treated with love and respect, so we project our version of that onto others. However, just below the surface where the dominant, most influential part of us resides, we are full of loathing, anger, and hatred for ourselves and others. We have just gotten so good at controlling that part that we are in a state of denial, doing all we can to suppress our rising anger levels and thoughts of suicide and revenge. It helps explain why people treat us the way they do, because it really does reflect back how we are treating ourselves (and others).

As counterintuitive as it may sound, regardless of what new technique you use to reprogram, control, or hide these thoughts and feelings, they will not go anywhere while we think they are not helpful to us. The more effort and technology we throw at fixing ourselves, the more we resemble a slow gas leak that is waiting for the spark to ignite it. The more we double down on fixing what isn't malfunctioning, the more our blame addiction is reflected back in increasingly intense ways through other people—all to show us what needs addressing and healing, so we can finally get to know who we honestly are and live a life of freedom, passion, and joy.

Imagining a Life Not Dominated by Blame

Have you ever thrown a ball with your nondominant hand? It just feels weird, so you very rarely practice improving it. In the same way, after your first Spanish for beginners class, you head to the bar to order your first beer. The closer you get to the bartender, the less you remember. "Beer please" comes out in your native tongue. It's just easier to keep doing what you always did.

When it comes to blame, it is a little more complicated because there hasn't been an alternative. You blame them or you blame yourself. We can't fathom a world where blame isn't our default reaction and control isn't our go-to solution. So we naturally reason that if we are responsible for co-creating the situations in our lives, and those situations are causing us mental and emotional pain, that must mean it is our fault, we F'd up, we are sabotaging ourselves.

Sara had bent over backwards during a proposal to give a client of hers everything they asked for. Extra references? Check. A second analysis of their quarterly numbers? No problem. A 10 percent discount and another week to make a decision? Sure thing.

She was devastated when, after all that work, the client went with a competitor. To add salt to the wound, she later found out they paid more and didn't receive the same perks she had offered. Based on her victim mentality this decision made no sense, so she blamed herself for not being good enough. She would *learn from her mistakes* and work even harder next time. She tried to let go and move on. She told herself, "Everything happens for a reason." However, the massive dose of self-blame remained intact. It was just hidden behind lots of self-help and motivational platitudes.

She was a successful businesswoman, but bitterness and resentment had built up over the years, which unknowingly impacted all her decisions—at work and in the home.

I said to Sara, "I know for a fact you didn't wholeheartedly want to work with this client." It wasn't the first time I'd had this conversation with her, which is why she replied with, "I knew you were going to say that. I have been getting self-honest. I know it is my fault, but I can't see why I would hold myself back. I really did want the client!" She concluded that she felt she had lost her mojo. She didn't realize as soon as she said, "I know it is my fault," and "hold myself back," she was in self-blame, and her insistence that she wanted to work with this particular client was keeping her from discovering the whole truth.

When we are in this self-blame mindset, any self-reflection will confirm our victim-infused questions. She was basically asking herself, "What did I do WRONG!" "Why do I keep sabotaging myself?" When this is the blame-based intention behind the self-enquiry, either no answer will arrive because nothing went wrong or you will hear confirmation that you made a mistake or failed. In this case, Sara received confirmation she had lost her mojo and wasn't a good salesperson anymore. She latched onto this, even though her history proved this was very far from reality. What actually happened was that more of her (again, even if it was 51 percent) didn't want to work with that type of client at this particular time. There was something she wasn't honestly happy with about the situation, but it was being covered up with all the self-blame and fake positive rhetoric.

To guide Sara through this part of the blame-recovery process, I repeated that I knew she wholeheartedly didn't want to work with that client at that time under the terms that were on the table. I was looking at the simple fact that she didn't win the client. I got her to write down the reasons she did want the client—money and prestige—so it would be out of her head. Then I had her write down a mirror list of all the things she didn't like about the client (and anyone else that came to mind). It wasn't long before some obvious similarities emerged in their characteristics and behaviors. A few made Sara chuckle as the reflection was so obvious now. Sara accused her client of "Being controlling," and "Always beating her down on price." Sara had a reputation as a control freak with her employees. And with her suppliers, she had a similar practice of doing all she could to knock down the price. The issue was, it had become a game of "I win, you lose," rather than good business practice.

As Sara went down her lists, she began to access her self-honesty. She collected all the evidence she needed to show her that if the client signed up, it would have actually caused her to lose money.

The fact is, she didn't lose her mojo or self-sabotage herself. Her honest truth was she didn't want to close this deal not only because it wasn't a profitable decision, but she also didn't have the employees to satisfy the client's needs—meaning, her industry leading reputation would be at risk. After admitting this to herself, she immediately felt relief. She realized that she genuinely got what she wanted. It wasn't the client who turned her down, it was an unconscious joint decision because their honest needs didn't match.

Playing the Blame Game is an effortful route to getting what we truly want. For Sara it came with excessive emotional pain. She was beating herself up for failing to close the deal. She had ventured into a maze looking for any perceived self-limiting belief and negative pattern like her ThetaHealer had told her to do. She became frustrated and depressed, as with every turn she concluded it was her fault.

Self-blame and the self-honesty it hides can also show up in the form of physical pain too. I had a client who came to me with a pain in his back that wouldn't go away regardless of what physical rehabilitation he tried. He injured his back a week prior to a stag weekend getaway with a bunch of his old college buddies. He lamented that the injury was his fault. He'd made a mistake by playing two rounds of golf after two years off. He expressed frustration because it prevented him from connecting with his friends.

Sensing there was more to the story, I asked him more about his life. He admitted that leading up to the injury, he'd made a commitment to get healthier. He started going to the gym several times per week and following a healthier diet. He reiterated that before the injury he was feeling great and looking forward to the weekend away with the boys.

After a few rounds of *I know for a fact you didn't want to go*, followed by a determined *yes I did*, he sighed and said, "Okay, if I'm going to be totally honest, I didn't really want to go. It was going to mess up my progress on my health. And plus, I really don't like where they are going."

Based on previous experience, if he admitted to these friends that he didn't want to go for this reason, they would guilt-trip him, and he would never hear the end of it. So, unconsciously it was easier to create an injury he could blame rather than confess that he didn't want to go. Indeed, his own ignorance made it even easier for him to convince *others* that his "bad luck" was the reason he couldn't go.

What can seem unbelievable is that our physical pain can disappear in the presence of self-honesty. But this is what regularly happens with my clients. This time was no different. As soon as he was honest about not wanting to go, his back pain disappeared. Why? Because he finally stopped blaming himself (and his back) for doing something wrong. He thought he had made a mistake by playing golf, when in fact it was an unconscious decision to help him get what he honestly wanted.

It can sound too simple, but it does take a whole new awareness to get to this simplicity. At times it can seem counterintuitive before it becomes intuitive, as the nuance of what is being offered can be passed off as just semantics. However, not is all as it may seem.

Learn from Your "Mistakes"

There is a lot of talk in the business world and in leadership training about treating our failures as opportunities to grow. We are supposed to learn from our mistakes so we can avoid repeating the same errors in the future. We are told to fail fast, fail often. You are not trying hard enough if you have never failed. Dare to fail if you want to succeed. It's okay to make mistakes; mistakes are our teachers; they help us learn. It sounds progressive and feels like we are taking control of our lives, but this mentality is just self-blame in disguise. It sounds empowering because it matches the growth mindset that we have been told is imperative to a happy and productive existence, but the subtext is self-blame—that we messed up.

It is our blame addiction that leads us to perceive our actions as "mistakes" when things don't pan out the way we anticipate, and it fuels the spinning of the Victim Cycle. It keeps our focus on "not making the same mistake" as opposed to focusing our energy on getting self-honest so we can honestly heal and find creative solutions.

A video-game designer was in the process of pitching his new fantasy-style role-playing idea to gaming publishers. He didn't have much experience in the boardroom but he was determined to learn. During his first meeting he tried to stay relaxed and came across as laid-back. The publishers didn't take on his project, and their feedback indicated that he was too lighthearted. They were concerned he wasn't reliable enough for a formal partnership. So, for his next meeting, he showed up in polished loafers and a nothing-but-business attitude. These publishers also turned him down, this time saying he seemed too stiff and not flexible enough to manage a design team. The cycle repeated itself, with the designer trying every which way to learn from his mistakes. Soon, he was left feeling like he would never succeed. He blamed the publishers for not wanting him, himself for not being good enough, and even his game idea for being subpar.

From my personal experience and after thousands of hours with clients, the "learn from your mistakes" mantra actually creates the very things it tries to avoid: that is, more situations and experiences that will be referred to as mistakes. Every round reflects back our diminishing self-esteem. The goal of correcting mistake after mistake is unsustainable, as we eventually run out of fixes. Businesses that adopt this strategy slowly lose their ability to empathize and either close down or become automated by introducing machines, AI, and robotics to limit the biggest cause of perceived mistakes—humans.

Deep in his blame addiction, the video-game designer also assumed the executives had all the decision-making power. In his narrative, they were the ones choosing or rejecting him. But at the very least, in any interaction it takes two to tango. Decisions are never one-sided even if it looks like it on the surface. What actually transpires is that our unconscious (self-honest) plan comes to fruition. Often in ways we can't imagine due the length of time we have been in a state of denial (or ignorance).

I got my client to self-reflect with different awareness. Rather than seeing each instance as a mistake (blame), I asked him to see it as an experience that mirrored back his self-honesty. He noticed how the executives' behaviors and comments gave valuable and honest self-reflection. In one particular company, their seemingly lack of interest reflected back his lack of passion for what they could offer him. Another executive, who he saw as rude and distracted, offered him an opportunity to see that he'd walked in the meeting in the same way. He thought he had covered up his frustration and ongoing financial issues with a hyper-fake positive exterior.

Because the game designer blamed himself for making what he saw as mistakes, he overlooked opportunities to become more self-honest. Like Sara, he did not honestly want to sign a deal at that time with these people. In some meetings, he unconsciously acted laid-back, not because he was sabotaging himself but because he didn't really want to work with the suit-and-tie-wearing corporate game publishers. Even when he met with companies he wanted to be associated with, he didn't actually want them to hire him as a freelancer. His honest desire was to become a permanent member of their staff. The combination of his unconscious dishonesty with himself and confusion about what he honestly wanted would have been interpreted by the executives as, "I don't know why, but I don't feel like this is the guy for us."

It's common to feel as though our thoughts, feelings, experiences, and behaviors are holding us back. There is a constant reminder from people in authority that we are "our own worst enemy" and our mind is doing all it can to "trick and sabotage us." It is laid on so thick that we feel like an outcast if we don't believe this blame-based narrative. In the previous chapter, Joan kept trying to correct the so-called mistakes her father made. She blamed him for her abandonment issues, which explained the reason why she had trouble finding a loving partner. It always resulted in more pain. That was until she got honest with herself about what she really wanted.

When self-blame is running the show, we come up with more blame-based fixes, like forming rigid habits.

What About My Bad Habits?

"I can't believe it!" clients frequently tell me as they engage with this recovery process. "Blame is everywhere!" And it is. Blame is present in nearly every conversation we have. One of the main things we often blame ourselves for is having bad habits. If only we could stop binge-watching Netflix every evening and start getting to the gym, we would be in great shape. If only we could stop dating assholes and start attracting sensitive guys, we would have a happy relationship. If only we could stop sleeping in until 9 a.m. and instead spring out of bed like the rest of the 5 a.m. club, we would be senior VP by now.

For many, self-blame is an endless tape reminding us how shitty we are. *If only I could shut my mind off! Why can't I just stop myself like others seem to do?* It is so relentless, it manages to feed a multibillion-dollar industry that gives us untold ways to forcibly change our mental and physical habits from what we deem as negative to something we think is positive. The whole approach has blame written all over it. We don't see it because of the confusing advice around self-blame. On one hand, you are told you should stop beating yourself up and love yourself instead. And on the other hand, you are told to blame yourself, as this is the way to take responsibility for your behavior—it's your fault; you only have yourself to blame.

What is it? Don't blame yourself because it isn't your fault, or do blame yourself because it is your fault! It mirrors the often contradictory messaging that is rampant in the self-development arena. There is a possibility blame doesn't even need to be part of the equation.

When blame isn't present, we no longer seek to replace our perceived bad habits and behaviors with what we consider good ones. Instead, we start to become aware of how everything is helping us on our journey to discover who we honestly are. And the closer we get to that by recovering from our blame addiction, the more our habits and behaviors will naturally change. No self-discipline or control is needed. Just like a client who told me that her twenty-year smoking habit vanished overnight. She didn't use willpower or techniques, she just woke up feeling disgusted by the idea of smoking. The main reason people smoke is to keep pushing down all the blame-based stories they have from the past. In my client's case, there was lots of anger towards her parents. When the blame and anger were no longer there, she no longer needed the necessary chemicals to turn the volume down.

Another client told me that he had unwittingly been sabotaging his progress in overcoming his fears and laziness. After reading a book, he decided to wake up at the crack of dawn to journal, work out, read, and meditate. It worked for a while, but he couldn't resist the temptation of the snooze button if he didn't get to bed at the time his evening routine dictated. To solve this, he hired a life coach. This helped a lot, as his coach preempted this and gave him a list of positive affirmations to recite as he woke up: "I will succeed today!" "I'm worthy of love." "I'm in charge of my life!" Brilliant. It worked. It got him to the kitchen where his bulletproof coffee was waiting. He was back on track.

But it was dependent on him being in one place for long periods of time. His perceived good habits were dependent on him having access to all his life hacks and conveniences. As soon as he traveled, worked late, or went out with friends, he needed an extreme amount of energy-intensive self-discipline to maintain the rigidity he had hired a coach to enforce.

It started to induce more fear and guilt. The fear of relapse forced him to get up when his mind and body were screaming at him to sleep more. On the occasions he listened, he felt guilty and more lazy! It got really frustrating when his new coach started telling him how important sleep was. And that this is the most important part of his day. While trying to please his new coach, he started to force himself to not go out, to not watch TV late, and to work out more.

He was doing everything right but couldn't understand why he was feeling more tired, getting ill more often, and not as motivated to promote his business. Feeling like a loser, he listened to more podcasts. Again, he suddenly felt better, but soon the frustration was back as his old perceived bad habits returned. It is a common scenario I hear often from my clients.

Being encouraged to divide your days into perceived good and bad habits is a symptom of our blame addiction. Whether the transition from bad to good is gradual or sudden is irrelevant because the change isn't sustainable simply because it is based on a false premise—we are doing something that isn't helping us, and it needs fixing.

If we look at the extreme end of the scale, we don't realize our addictions are helping to keep us alive, not kill us. Someone doesn't shoot up heroine because they are happy. We don't get paralytic to the point we forget what we did the night before because we are enjoying life. We are deeply unhappy and the drug of choice is giving us time. Time to heal. The issue is, we haven't known how to self-heal so we keep borrowing time wherever we can.

Blaming ourselves for having so-called bad habits keeps us in the Victim Cycle. It numbs us to the ever-changing subtle and obvious messages that we are receiving. Maybe today our body wants green tea instead of bulletproof coffee. Perhaps our body is asking for limes instead of lemons. Or I may even be ingesting too much vitamin D for the time of year. Maybe our lack of sleep is because we are blaming ourselves or others in our past. We won't know until we exit the Victim Cycle and get better at honestly listening to ourselves.

Thinking that our habits are holding us back makes sense. It is the path of least resistance to think this way, like it is for shopaholics to pop out and get that much-needed pair of shoes on payday. Beating yourself up for not having enough self-control is an easy way to get your blame fix. At the beginning, when the self-deprecating thoughts gave you fuel to get up at 5 a.m. or you could replace them with their positive alternative, you liked it. But when all the stored-up blame hits you at once and something unexpected happens that you think is bad, you don't leave bed because the covers feel like a protective shield hiding you from the unfair world outside.

This is why learning even better ways to develop self-control so we can stick to our rigid habits feels good. It feels amazing to have a cold shower. You feel alive. Before you know it, your new ice bath isn't quite hitting the spot, so you invest in a trip to jump in an ice-covered lake. It takes you beyond what you thought possible. You appreciate the serenity as the internal chatter is silenced for a while. But what are these approaches to life teaching you? They show you how incredible the human mind and body are, that is for sure. They might even temporarily reduce inflammation as a result. But they are also keeping you in the control-and-conquer mindset, confirming your honest thoughts are bad and you must do what you can to ignore them. It keeps you in the Victim Cycle. It keeps you jumping from one addiction to another.

Just as any technique to control ourselves isn't the enemy, cold therapy isn't either. It is a way to tick something we deem as positive off our list and feel in control of our day. This is all we have known. After all, if we allowed ourselves to go with whatever felt good, wouldn't we just eat ice cream and watch *Gladiator* all day in our pajamas? Or wouldn't a heroin addict just shoot up at every possible opportunity? Nobody would ever go to work!

I am not saying, "Just do what feels right." A serial killer would continue to murder people if you advised them to do whatever they love to do or to follow their passion. What I am saying is: these concerns of spiraling into a pit of despair and gluttony are coming from a foundation steeped in blame addiction. It is why they do happen and why we use these instances as evidence that more control is needed.

We often eat ice cream or shoot up heroin because we are blaming our parents for messing us up or our siblings for not being there when we most needed them. We talk about "comfort food" and make jokes about eating gallons of ice cream after a breakup because binging on these foods is a way to numb the pain. The same is true of habitual drug use, which is often seen as a sign of deep trauma. It's a way to run away and hide. But again, hide from what? Where is the pain originating from? With less blame, there is less pain.

Habits are barometers letting us know something needs addressing. They reflect back how much blame, victimhood, and fear is in our foundation. The idea is for our habits and behaviors to naturally change as we heal. Sticking to rigid habits might enable us to afford a new sports car or condo, but it is one of the prevailing reasons the deep feeling of honest joy and happiness is so elusive and transitory.

Habits Are Barometers

Is life really as simple as classing one habit as good and one as bad? Isn't life a little more nuanced than that?

Habits are barometers to what is going on in our lives, and once we no longer dichotomize them, they can help us get more honest with ourselves. For instance, maybe we see our overweight coworker, Nigel, bent over his computer every day hunch-shouldered and ashen-faced. Do we think to ourselves that his problem is hunched shoulders? Does he simply need to get in the habit of sitting up straighter or go to the gym?

Probably not! More likely we'd think, *Now there's a sad chap* or *Ask if he's okay*. Nigel's habit of stooping over is an indicator to show us that something within him needs addressing. The habit isn't a problem, it's a sign that can lead us to a deeper understanding of ourselves if we listen to it in a different way.

It is no secret that we are living in a time that demands instant gratification. Our self-help advice is no different. What is the quickest way to get out of a funk and into a positive mind-set? Maybe you tried meditating for twenty minutes twice a day while reciting a mantra. That didn't work or took too long, so you went shopping. Become more confident in two minutes with a power pose—sold! But surely there is something quicker. How about five seconds. Just interrupt any self-doubt and negative talk with a high five and you can break any bad habit.

Does Nigel really need more ways to control and push away his self-honesty? Or is he unconsciously crying out for some deep and honest healing?

No amount of trips to the gym, forcing his shoulders back, or investing in the latest ergonomic furniture is going to be a long-term solution. Nigel is screaming out for honest healing. His body has been talking to him for a while. He is contracting. His back is rounded and shoulders rolled forward, unconsciously trying to find comfort in the fetal position he deep down remembers. The side effect of recovering from our blame addiction is that our posture automatically changes to match our newfound confidence. After, we naturally feel taller and lighter as the burden of blame lifts from our shoulders. To get to this point, we have to learn how to honestly listen to our thoughts and body rather than trying to shut them up or separate ourselves from them.

The Habit of Self-Blame

Clients tell me how frustrated they are after years of trying to control the self-blame swirling around in their mind: "I feel I am a piece of shit!" "I am not worthy!" "I feel I am not good enough." "I hate myself!" So I understand why any "positive habit" or new quick technique is eagerly consumed just to feel better and take the pain away.

When a client comes to me looking to lose weight, for example, they will expect me to give them exercise and nutrition habits to follow. Instead, I take them on the honest healing process and wait for them to tell me they "just didn't feel like eating chocolate today." Or, "It has been a week, and I have gone for a walk every day." It is often followed by a surprising comment that it was so effortless. Long-term fears, phobias, and addictions have also effortlessly disappeared following the same process because the underlying reason for their cravings has been addressed—our blame addiction.

One client went out for a cigarette during our session. He came back, sat down, and proceeded to chug an entire glass of water. Then he turned to me and said, "That was very strange. I took one drag of my cigarette, coughed my guts up, and threw it away. And that was the best-tasting water I've ever had!"

His body responded like it did the first time he smoked over thirty years before. It didn't want the thousands of chemicals it contained then, and it didn't want them now. The difference was that he had exited the Victim Cycle during our session and he no longer needed to consume something that helped him push away his blame-based (self-deprecating) thoughts *because they were not there anymore.*

During our corporate programs, we get the participants to stand up and "check in." We ask them to simply scan and connect to their body with their mind's eye and listen. They might have never done anything like this exercise before, but the large majority report how much better they feel. Energy levels increase and pain and tension can lesson. They are often surprised. But it isn't miraculous. It is just the first time many people have actually had a break from ignoring and blaming their body and honestly listened in a blame-free space.

CHAPTER 10

Uncomfortable Levels of Self-Honesty

For too many years to imagine, we have been blaming something for why we think our life isn't going the way it should. On an esoteric level, God, fallen angels, spirits, demons, and the universe have been made scapegoats. Of course, parents, siblings, partners, and bosses are next in line. But nothing gets more blame than our brain and mind. As many things as there are to blame, there are also approaches that promise to transform any "bothersome" thought, pattern, and belief into life-changing positive ones. We have moved from electroshock therapy and lobotomies to psychoanalysis, medication, hypnosis, and other intensive techniques all designed to help us remove, unearth, reprogram, and delete anything we deem as "holding us back."

Doubling down on finding ways to fix our physical brain and eradicate the perceived negative chatter it contains is resulting in more pain, not less. If this was the answer and we had so many ways of achieving this goal, wouldn't we see a decrease in mental and physical illness? Why are we still experiencing an increase in suicide, civil unrest, and economic hardship? We are told more research is needed to unpack the inner workings of the mind and brain. But if all that research is based on the same blame-based premise that something is broken and hell-bent on being a constant hindrance in our lives, we will always get the same blame-based fixes.

I became a little suspicious of this *our mind and brain are out to get us* line of thinking the more clients I saw. I realized that two people with the same thoughts and beliefs can have completely different outcomes. It dawned on me that, like everything else, the issue isn't with the *thing*—the thought, belief, pattern, or limbic brain that needs our attention; it is with our foundation and what it is made of. Our foundation is what influences how we perceive events and the decisions that result.

Twin brothers could live in the same house, with the same parents, and go to the same school. They could have the same belief that money is the root of all evil and think they are stupid and have low self-esteem. Why does one grow up to be a millionaire and the other ends up on welfare? They can walk into a driving test, both *believing* they'll fail it, and yet one could pass and the other won't. Why? It isn't because they are not visualizing enough or that one has so-called unconscious self-limiting beliefs. It is because one honestly doesn't want to pass. One might want to be able to drive so he can have a peaceful commute to work in the city, while the other doesn't because he secretly enjoys spending quality time with mom while he gets a ride to work.

After a lifetime of doing our best to avoid self-honesty and controlling our "inner demons," we might not like what we find when we start listening. It can feel really uncomfortable. Every cell of our body might want to do what it has always done, such as quickly put on an uplifting song or podcast or watch a motivational video. Sometimes this helps quell the anger, sadness, or worry. Sometimes not. Our experience might be that any quiet time you have is unbearable due to the internal dialogue detailing every which way your friend was horrible, unsupportive, and mean to you.

Looking for any respite, your body helps you out. You might not see it this way because you feel intense, chronic fatigue and lethargy. Where not even your favorite song or podcaster can keep you awake. But sleep is where the noise stops. That is until nightmares invade your last refuge. It is not a nice image or feeling, but I knew it well in my life and in that of my clients.

Finding new and improved ways to hide, block, and control our self-honesty seems like the skill we need to improve. But actually, it is learning to listen. Not in a way we have been used to while "meditating" or using other mindfulness practices. Rather, listening with a brand-new awareness while being in a state of blame-free connection, curiosity, and imagination.

Better Out Than In

When the noise and pain become too much, you might seek help from an anger management retreat or a couple's therapy session. You leave feeling lighter because you have gotten stuff off your chest. You are encouraged to talk things out from now on rather than bottle it up. Armed with various tools and techniques to facilitate healthy communication, you feel optimistic. Better out than in, right? As you leave the parking lot, you give it a go. Standing in your power, you express your newfound honesty, only to find yourself minutes later saying, "Don't get angry with me; I am only being honest."

Being encouraged to talk things out sounds good on paper. And of course it has its time and place. However, when the people involved are unknowingly addicted to blame, it becomes a victim fest. All that comes out is blame diarrhea— sometimes in overt ways where it resembles a shoot-out at the O.K. Corral. Other times it is subtle and passive aggressive, like two grand-master chess players each expertly maneuvering their points around the topic looking for checkmate. I'm right, you're wrong. This can all be averted when we focus on being honest with ourselves first before diving in and being honest with others.

If we keep it simple, two things can result when we focus on being honest with ourselves first. We don't need to talk to the person anymore because we finally realize that the person we are annoyed with is actually mirroring back our own gripes and insecurities about ourselves. And if we do talk to them, it will be well received with no defenses up because there is no blame being thrown around.

It was an uncomfortable eureka moment for a client of mine who realized his wife wasn't actually the enemy he portrayed her to be. For years he had blamed his wife for starting every argument, especially the ones they had in the car. He realized there were times he just wanted to be in the car on his own. He loved the freedom of stopping when he wanted and singing as loud as he could with the window down. These were all things his wife complained about. He recognized how he became more sensitive and argumentative when he wanted to be alone. Because he was blaming her for being the reason he couldn't do what he wanted, anytime he asked for some space it resulted in conflict. So he learned to suck it up, bite his tongue, and walk on eggshells. Which inevitably led to more arguments.

After getting self-honest, he was able to speak to his wife with no blame in the air. This was the first time he had ever done this. He couldn't believe how effortless their conversations had become. Because blame wasn't reverberating around the car and bouncing off the walls at home, his wife was able to be more honest also and confessed there were times she preferred to drive alone. The fear of upsetting each other disappeared. And even more surprisingly, they actually started to enjoy more time together, not less. Ultimately, the issue had to do with their blame addiction and not them having time alone in the car.

Playing in the Blame Game for as long as we have leads to excessive mental, emotional, and physical pain. The recovery process can also come with discomfort. But this is only because of the way we have been using control, acceptance, and dishonesty to achieve healing.

Self-Blame vs. Self-Honesty

Media conglomerates, politicians, tech companies, and Big Pharma, are accused of propaganda and spreading misinformation. Religions are blamed for starting wars. Weapons manufacturers are the reason we have school shootings. As true and unquestionable as these may seem to be, they are not the reason we do what we do. Everyone is exposed to the same weapons, propaganda, and religious and philosophical dogma (and jokes), but it is how we individually perceive them that impacts us and how we behave. Even hypnotists are happy to confirm that not everyone can be hypnotized.

I am not defending the actions of these institutions; I have lots of ideas about how the world could run more peacefully. What I am saying is: there is a way we can profoundly heal as individuals that will have a profound ripple impact on the whole. If we keep thinking *they* are the ones that have to change, we are once again fulfilling Einstein's definition of insanity.

If it isn't them and it isn't us and our thoughts that are holding us back—then what is?

Taking any opportunity to confirm our victimhood keeps us in the belief that life is full of hardships, barriers, and blocks to overcome. It is a painful and exhausting way to live, especially when we resort to the only solution we have known—to double down on our positive thinking and use any tools and techniques we have to control and conquer any emotional or physical pain we experience.

But what if nothing is holding us back? What if we are always helping ourselves?

Colin thought this was a crazy idea, as he was incredibly frustrated after our first few sessions. "It's not working!" he exclaimed. "The pain in my body is still preventing me from doing what I want. The Universe is stopping me. It looks like I am relegated to a life of chronic fatigue and autoimmune disorders." Even though Colin was a life coach and spent over ten years learning the latest neuroscience-backed healing and transformation modalities, he told me his mental and physical health had been in rapid decline for the last five years. His annoyance was further fueled by the fact his mother recommended me. Colin couldn't understand why she got results so soon when he knew so much more about healing—not realizing what he actually knew was more ways to blame and control than his mother did.

As much as Colin thought he was putting my philosophy into practice, he was doubling down on what he knew. Colin's case was a little more complicated than others because he had a business that was built on his teachings. It is like a person who is dependent on their disease or injury to keep collecting state benefits or handouts from family. They are invested in staying the same, as their livelihood is dependent on their pain remaining. It is not that Colin didn't want to change; it is that he had a lot of cognitive biases that he needed to prove right by proving me wrong. In short, everything I was offering him was in direct conflict with the blame and control-based teaching he had spent a lot of time and money learning. I was fully empathetic with Colin, as I had been in exactly the same situation, spending thousands on learning the same things.

Colin's rebuttal—that he *was* being self-honest—was backed up with a list of his known issues and patterns. He had been working on them for years with lots of different people and modalities. *I honestly hate myself and what I am doing and where I live. My father hit me a lot when I was a child and often locked me in my room for hours.* Colin told me, "I feel like I am being honest, but nothing is changing…I'm just reliving past *negative* memories and rehashing old shit again."

There is a difference between being self-honest and confirming your victimhood. Colin had more work to do. He was beating himself up for not "getting it." It was like being disappointed you don't know how to order a full dinner for the family in Spanish after a few language lessons. Colin was very much in the Victim Cycle after years of dedicated study—each modality reaffirmed his past was bad, his parents "fucked him up," his brain kept malfunctioning regardless of how much he followed their teachings and *retrained his faulty wiring*. He had accepted every label he had ever been given. And what's more, he was ingraining this way of thinking as he was teaching it to his clients.

Colin was getting better at self-blame, not at being self-honest. Even though he could accurately claim he was being honest when he stated his hatred for himself and his job, that isn't being *self-honest* about his contribution in co-creating his situation.

The basics of getting more self-honest come down to exploring the possible ways in which we contributed to an experience. For example, when a friend cancels dinner plans at the last minute you might ask, *Did I contribute in any way?* This question is easy to answer depending on how much you have exercised your creative and perception muscle. If you are in the blame mindset, the answer is an easy no: you will accuse them of being flaky, rude, or inconsiderate regardless of the situation. When you are being self-honest, you are in a state of curiosity. You know there is a possibility you had something to contribute and pose the question, *Did I wholeheartedly want to go out with that person, at that time, at that venue?*

We have explored this idea in previous examples but it is worth reiterating as our blame defenses can shoot off when we feel like a "wrong" has been committed. Maybe we wanted to stay in and look after our new puppy. Or we have only three more episodes to go on our latest boxset binge. It might be raining, there might be a pandemic, your haircut didn't go as planned, you have a pimple. There are so many possibilities to entertain.

If you are disappointed, mad, or angry with your friend, then it is an indication that you are in blame. If you are connecting with your emotions and body in a curious way, then you are engaging with your self-honesty.

You might become aware that your accusations of them being flaky and rude are traits that might relate to you more than you would like to admit. You might want to use this opportunity to make them feel really bad so you can use it as an excuse to not go to their wedding. Even if you don't come up with many possible contributions, the fact you entered this curious mindset will be beneficial because it means you were out of the Victim Cycle. And the more you do this, the less you will find yourself in it.

I have worked with dancers and actors who have prepared weeks in advance for an audition only to not get the part, not realizing that their priorities changed before the big audition. They met a new partner and wanted to spend time with them rather than go on tour or be on set for an extended time. Some have admitted to a long list of fears and insecurities that would have contributed to why they didn't honestly want to get the gig, like the actress who had no problem getting work on stage but never got callbacks for TV or film work. After a while it became apparent that she was self-conscious about her weight. There is a well-known meme in the industry that the "camera puts on ten pounds," and this often played on her mind. However, when we got really honest, it wasn't any of her fears or insecurities that stopped her or "blocked" her from getting these jobs, it was that she didn't honestly want to work in front of the camera. She loved stage work. She loved the history and the fact it was live. I helped her realize that maybe she didn't have as many fears as she thought, and that her self-confidence wasn't low, as these didn't show up when she was on stage doing what she honestly loved.

Feeling Your Way to Freedom

Getting self-honest is also about *feeling*. And that ability comes with practice.

I gave Colin instructions to sit or lie down and listen to his body. He told me his heart was beating really fast. The story of the day rattled around in his mind. His brother had chewed him out and criticized him. He wanted it to just stop. Instead, I asked him to tell me where he felt the discomfort in his body: "My legs, hands, and jaw." Colin had been trained to see his thoughts as negative and either transform them into positive alternatives, or observe them in the hope they would pass on by. To help him out of this blame approach, I guided Colin to let each thought and body part know he was listening to them. While in this state I asked him to remember, based on his new awareness he had gotten from our work together, that his thoughts were helping him find out where he held emotions in his body so he could honestly heal. All his body wanted was to be listened to with a curious mindset.

It took over an hour for him to settle, as the self-blame record was caught in a groove because he kept trying to control and push his thoughts and emotions away. Then all of a sudden, the needle shifted and the beat changed. Not in a positive or upbeat way, but in a way that felt like an altered state. At that point I asked him to once again place 100 percent focus on any part of his body that was talking to him. Being in this altered state, he was able to feel, listen, and observe in a very different way than how he had ever done previously.

Colin, like most of us, had been proactively doing all he could to heal with the control- and blame-based tools that were available to him. As such, his focus had been to get rid of the pain, not realizing this was self-blame. It can sound crazy that all the time we are wanting our pain to go, it will actually remain, requiring ever more powerful drugs or other intervention to numb it. All of Colin's teachings and coaching sessions reinforced that his mind, body, and brain were separate and doing something wrong. During our sessions, his pain effortlessly left as a by-product of being in this curious listening space. But it would soon return as the days unfolded—as he reverted back to his blame- and control-based teachings.

It can seem a strange idea that all our mental, emotional, and physical pain are helping us when the mainstream wisdom is telling us otherwise. Colin's mind remained closed to this idea, and I couldn't help him in the time we had together.

Stepping outside our comfort zones to come face-to-face with our self-honesty can be uncomfortable at first. But the intense feelings are nothing compared to the slow, drawn-out pain that comes with our control-based strategies: denial, acceptance, and avoidance.

As one client commented, "Thank you again for helping me honestly listen. I love it not only because life is easier and more fun this way, but because I enjoy exploring what my honesty actually is. I am getting to know myself in a new and different way. I see more clearly now that honoring how I truly feel, though it takes practice, is rewarding because it allows for unapologetic honesty once fear of the truth fades away. And it brings forth only one thing, which is Love."

Pain Is a Blessing in Disguise

There are a number of areas that get a lot of pushback in regards to my philosophy; that we have some contribution to make to our experiences, and that our contribution is ultimately helping us. Infertility and miscarriage are two that can seem incomprehensible. Of course, for some couples it is understandable because they have admitted that they never wanted children. But for couples who believe they wholeheartedly want children, it is very painful news. Especially when they are given a number of medical or psychological labels that explain their circumstance.

My confidence that not only do we have a contribution that helps us, based on our unknown honest motivations, but that any label can be reversed, comes from my near 100 percent success rate for helping couples conceive when they were told it was impossible. The only time my clients didn't give birth is when they discovered the hidden, but honest, reasons they really didn't want children. After helping a couple have their first child, they came back to me wanting help with their second. After many months with little success, they reasoned, it worked the first time so maybe it will work again.

This couple were deeply in love, but the pressure of their first child had taken its toll. They had always agreed they wanted two or three to feel like a complete family. So, even though they were experiencing emotional and financial pressure, they decided to try for a second child anyway, not realizing that a second child would have very probably been the straw that broke the camel's back in their relationship. They were at a teetering point. Deep down they knew this, but pushed it away and used every ounce of control they could muster to keep their "stuff" at bay, long enough to do the mechanical action to have a child. Once I took them through the blame-recovery process, their relationship radically improved; the laughter returned along with the joy of sex. Months later I received this message:

> *"I'm writing to let you know that we recently have a healthy daughter—born 17th September, weighing in at a healthy 8 lb 4 ozs and now spending most of the time clamped to Anna, feeding away! We wanted to thank you so much for the help you gave us in helping Amy come into this world— speaking to you at the tail end of last year really helped us realign ourselves…"*

Another couple came to see me after having a number of miscarriages. I asked them, "Do you want a baby at this time?" And they both enthusiastically responded, "Yes, we do." Based on my simple approach to life, I knew this wasn't the whole truth because they didn't have a baby. I also knew, as with many other couples I had helped give birth after similar experiences, the pain of each loss had worn away at their soul. I offered to my clients that our conscious plans are often in conflict with our deep self-honesty, so we co-create painful experiences to once again encourage us to honestly self-reflect so we can experience what we wholeheartedly want.

In their case, the husband had recently lost two jobs and had just started his third. As much as they wanted a baby, they had financial concerns and knew they might not be able to manage. They were doing what they had been told to do—"Just focus on the positive and everything will be fine. What is meant to be will be."

It is well documented that stress can stop a woman from having her period for months. Stress can bring on a heart attack. A person who has been in a relationship for decades can die of a broken heart when their partner dies. They quickly deteriorate as they manifest a fatal illness. My father became a common statistic when he followed a similar phenomenon—he died six months after he retired at the age of seventy. Whether it is a partner or a job, when something important is no longer there, you can lose your reason for living. It plays into the science of the *placebo* and *nocebo* effect.

It can be incredibly uncomfortable to think we had something to do with a miscarriage when we think we 100 percent want to give birth. As I mentioned, some clients don't need to hear my philosophy as they have come to their own conclusions. They can admit they were incredibly unsure and scared about having a baby so it wasn't a surprise when they miscarried. Others wished for it to happen. Each couple had the same experience but each had a different perspective and awareness that brought pain or relief with it.

Uncomfortable Levels of Self-Honesty

We are not used to getting uncomfortably honest in a world that is hyper-fake and "positive." We are encouraged to stay away from this part of us because we are told it is "negative" and we should control it. But this is the part of us that needs our attention. My philosophy can see defenses go up, but it is this approach that has helped so many couples give birth when they have been told it is impossible. It is this philosophy that has helped so many broken hearts find reason to carry on living.

We don't fully appreciate the impact our blame addiction has had on us. Our levels of ignorance and denial are high. This results in the literal and figurative calcification of our mind and body. It is why we often require extreme pain to get into the walnut where our honest self resides. If we were outside of the Victim Cycle, we wouldn't need extreme measures to help us find out and achieve what we honestly want. But all the while we are in the washing machine, we get numb to the subtle signs and must wait for the sledgehammer to arrive before we are jolted out of our shell.

There have been many times where athletes have injured themselves before an important match. This can sometimes occur during competition, like the example of UK sprinter Derek Redmond, who participated in the 1992 Olympic Games in Barcelona, Spain. During the semifinal of the 400-meter race he pulled a hamstring, thus dashing his long-held dreams of winning a medal. At the time, Derek felt searing pain and watched his competitors sprint past him, and I'm sure not one part of him was consciously wondering if this was a blessing in disguise.

Like most elite athletes, Derek put his heart and soul into getting to the Olympics. The pressure he put on himself was high; he didn't want to let the British people down, but mostly he didn't want to disappoint his father, who had sacrificed so much to get him to that point.

The path of least resistance would be to suggest that Derek had "bad luck" or didn't prepare correctly. However, without our blame blinkers on and the benefit of hindsight, we can see that there was more at play. Halfway down the track Derek knew he wasn't going to win and, in fact, wasn't going to finish very high in the race. Quicker than a quantum processor, he unconsciously undertook a risk analysis and concluded that an injury was the best option if he was to ultimately reach his honest dream of *notoriety* and making his father *proud*. As it is happening, it can seem strange to even contemplate that this moment would be the catalyst for him achieving what he honestly wanted.

As his hamstring snapped, Derek must have felt his world come to an end. At that moment, mixed emotions filled the stadium. The race was over and the winners were celebrating their victory as a broken man with a broken dream looked on halfway down the track. Derek stood up and proceeded to hobble in excruciating physical and emotional pain toward the finish line. He was unaware that an iconic Olympic memory was unfolding. The claps and cheers of encouragement built into a deafening crescendo as everyone realized what was happening. Everyone was on their feet as the world's commentators were cheering him on. We were all witnessing one of the greatest moments in sports as it gloriously epitomized the Olympic spirit that "it's the taking part that matters, not the winning."

The spectacle wasn't over. Suddenly, everyone's attention shifted to Derek's father, Jim, who broke protocol and made his way over to his son. Pushing past officials, he cradled Derek and became his crutch for the last hundred meters. Time stood still as Derek and Jim crossed the finish line together and history was made. Derek might not have been successful in his conscious goal of standing on the podium, but he did achieve his honest goal and unconscious endgame of becoming an iconic athlete at the Olympics and making his father and the British public proud.

Derek achieved the main goal, just not in the way he was attached to.

My interpretation becomes more plausible when we unpack more of Derek's life. We later found out that he'd always wanted to represent England in three sporting areas, which he later went on to achieve. It's fair to say that, if Derek finished fifth, sixth, or seventh in that Olympic sprint, he wouldn't have received the unrivaled adulation, publicity, and later career opportunities that he did. Even if he stood on the podium at the Olympics, he might have felt pressured to focus on track and field rather than achieve his other goals of representing England in basketball and motorsport.

Our minds and bodies are seamlessly interlinked. Eventually our self-honesty will always come to the surface in the form of thoughts, behaviors, feelings, or physical afflictions.

These moments of self-honesty aren't always fun. In fact, they can often be gut-wrenching. They can feel like thousands of years of ancestral pain is being listened to and healed. And yet, there is an unrecognizable sense of profound freedom that follows. The key is to get to the point where we are comfortable walking around perceiving events without our blame blinkers and blame-tinted glasses on. We start to enjoy *feeling* our experiences rather than trying to work out and understand them. This is true freedom.

Your Self-Honesty Influences Every Decision

There is enough psychology research to fill a football stadium. We have mountains of literature detailing all aspects of human behavior. It is mind-bending to contemplate all the possible reasons behind why we do what we do. Over the years, I have realized that much of it enforces our blame addiction rather than helps us heal from it. With that said, it has an important purpose. If you want to analyze human behavior for market-ing, entertainment, and manipulation purposes, then it is very useful. However, deep psychological analysis often confuses a simple process when it comes to profound and long-term heal-ing and transformation.

Our deep self-honesty and honest motivations have an impact on every decision we make, from who we marry to the career we pursue to what we watch on Netflix. The better we become at being truly honest with ourselves, the better we'll get at identifying our motivations. What I mean is: it is easy to beat yourself up for procrastinating or being lazy for not finishing your presentation prep. But your self-blame is actu-ally a dishonest act. When a high-performing executive came to me looking for help with his procrastination, I told him he was actually being very productive and efficient; he just didn't know what his honest motivation was for spending hours on social media when he should be preparing the accounts for his clients.

For him, his unconscious honest goal was to avoid his wife. They had been swirling around in the Victim Cycle, arguing with each other for months. It was exhausting. He had found it less stressful to avoid her by working late than it was to have another uncomfortable encounter. Based on his blame-based endgame—avoidance—-he unconsciously managed his day perfectly.

We don't need to know the specifics of where our thoughts, beliefs, or feelings originate from in order to heal. We don't need to blame our dating problems on how Mom and Dad treated us at age four. We don't need to pin our insecurities on our middle-school gym teacher. We don't need an OCD diagnosis to explain our obsessive thoughts. And we don't need drugs or therapies to change our thoughts and feelings from negative to positive. This whole approach keeps our blame addiction well fed.

We have accepted the idea that we have a separate part of our mind called the "subconscious" full of limiting beliefs, self-sabotaging patterns, and negative thoughts that hold us back. We have accepted that our minds somehow trick us into making the wrong decision and doing the wrong thing. But if we gain access to our self-honesty, we realize we're not actually making the wrong decisions at all, as they are all taking us toward what we honestly want—so we can honestly heal.

This was perfectly illustrated by Franz, who made his way through over a dozen interviews for a high-ticket position at a prestigious tech company. A year after getting the news that he was unsuccessful, Franz was still deep in his disappointment and depression. He was doing a good job of beating himself up for failing. It was vexing for him to hear, "I know for a fact you didn't wholeheartedly want the job." He looked at me like I just insulted his mother on the playground. With a little investigation it became obvious to me what his honest motivations were. He was newly married at the time with their first child on the way. The company had repeated many times how he would be "married" to the job. He knew it was going to be a demanding role, and Franz said all the right things to get to the final interview.

I said to him, "As much as you performed perfectly to get to the final stage, you also performed perfectly to not get the job." After a very uncomfortable thirty minutes as we discussed the possible ways he helped himself by not getting the job, he acknowledged how much he wanted to be around for his wife and first child. He was blaming his father for neglecting the family when he was a baby, so he vowed to not do the same. Franz's disappointment and depression lifted almost immediately upon admitting to himself that his overriding priority was to be there for his family and not the tech company.

I let him know that his emotional state, which had impacted every aspect of his life and health over the last year, stemmed from him being dishonest with himself. That was it. It wasn't his father's absence as a child or any self-sabotaging thoughts or behaviors. He was lying to himself that he wholeheartedly wanted the job, when more of him wanted to provide for his family in a different way. When he held his child for the first time, all his priorities changed. He felt the difference, but he controlled this because that is what we are trained to do. Focus on your goals and never give up. How could he after so many interviews and so much time invested?

The things we perceive as problems in our lives are not the whole story. We unconsciously co-create these painful situations with the people around us to achieve our true goals. We get emotional because our blame blinkers tame our curiosity to find out or listen to all the information, awareness, and wisdom that is available to us.

Our mind, body, and soul are super intelligent and interconnected with all other beings. Somehow this wisdom has been superseded by the idea our mind, body, and soul are stupid and isolated. This has taught us to ignore the very thing that is constantly talking to us, and doing all it can to help us achieve more than we think is possible.

Do You Like Being Ignored?

It is fair to say being ignored can be one of the most painful places to find yourself. It doesn't even need to be while we wait to hear back from our blind date the night before or for a client to sign an important contract. It can be your friend looking at their phone during dinner as you are telling them about your promotion. Being ignored can feel horrible. What about being ignored after you have been blamed for doing something wrong (which you know you didn't)? How does that feel? It can make people crazy.

Being on the receiving end of the silent treatment can be one of the most painful spaces to be. Most people know this feeling and the stress and tension it creates. Just watch a child desperately trying to get their parents' attention while they finally have five minutes to themselves. The child starts to act out, be naughty, and annoying just to be acknowledged. Why is it, then, that even though we are so familiar with this horrible feeling, we constantly give our mind and bodies the silent treatment? We blame them for doing things wrong and then do all we can to ignore and shut them up.

Self-healing can be simple and effortless. We have the innate potential to self-heal instantly. But we have to do something radically different to what we have been doing. And that is to start engaging with our mind and body (and environment) in a very different way rather than keep blaming and ignoring them.

Do you remember the toy Etch A Sketch? You could draw on it with two dials and then shake it and the slate would be clean for you to draw another picture. It was a great invention long before computers became mainstream. When we are in pain, we often want to shake ourselves or wave a magic wand and have all the pain disappear so we can get back to normal. However, that is the issue. The pain arrived because of whatever our normal was comprised of. Jake, an avid runner, came to me with an ankle pain. I asked him, "If I could click my fingers and your pain would vanish, what would you do?" With a big smile he confirmed my suspicions that he would celebrate with a 10K run.

When pain becomes too intense or it stops us from doing what we normally do, our focus narrows in on getting rid of the pain as quickly as possible. Jake was in this place. He was frustrated, not realizing he was blaming his ankle for doing something wrong and ignoring it. This can seem intuitive, and it is as if we are in a serious life-or-death situation. Stopping the bleeding and administering morphine, antihistamine, or an adrenaline shot can take away pain and save a life. Jake was not in this situation. He was attempting to make the pain go away, not realizing he wasn't listening to what it had to say. This is one of the main reasons the pain remains (or moves around the body), even if we are able to temporarily hide or subdue it.

Mental, emotional, and physical pain are all wrapped up together. They all show up at different times to offer signs, messages, and guidance. My goal for Jake was to shift his focus. Instead of getting rid of the pain, I wanted him to open a channel of communication with his ankle and the emotional pain he felt. I explained that for long-term and wide-reaching healing and transformation to take place, we want the pain to leave as a by-product of us getting better at listening to it. Too simple, right? Well, like any skill it takes practice before it becomes intuitive and effortless.

Jake looked me square in the eye and said, "Bullshit!" "With the most respect," he added.

Obviously still curious, Jake came back a year later with a diagnosis of "frozen shoulder." He'd had it for six months by the time he saw me, and none of the conventional methods had helped get rid of the pain. He was still in the same *blame and shame* and *ignore* mindset. He was blaming his stiff, painful shoulder joint for stopping him from doing his normal activities like playing golf, wakeboarding, and working on his entrepreneurial projects. But, like all of us, Jake was unknowingly addicted to blame. He didn't realize he was deep in his victimhood. By the end of the session, he was pain-free and frantically waving his hand over his head looking for the pain. During that session I didn't touch him at all or have him do any physical exercises. I didn't lobotomize his brain or use any rewiring, reprogramming, or hypnosis techniques.

How is this possible? How could he self-heal so quickly after his doctor, physiotherapist, and personal trainer said he would need another six to twelve months of physical rehabilitation before he would gain any semblance of pain-free movement? Timing is important. He was definitely more ready than the first time. However, after guiding him to explore possible ways in which his symptoms were helping him get what he honestly wanted, he repeatedly assured me that the pain and discomfort were in no way helping him with anything, let alone getting in touch with his honest motivations. He categorically affirmed that it was an inconvenience, as he couldn't play golf wakeboard or finish some of his entrepreneurial projects.

I focused on freeing him from his attachment to his label. He had seen X-rays and MRIs so he had proof—when in fact he just had proof to show what blame does to the human body. As he stepped outside the Victim Cycle for a moment, he said, "Truth be told, because I couldn't do any of my normal stuff, I found myself spending more time with my eldest son." And there it was: his deep self-honest priority. His shoulder pain, discomfort, and inconvenience were all there to help him reach this awareness.

Profound healing doesn't always happen this quickly, but at that moment, when he accessed his honest motivation to spend time with his son, he relaxed. I could feel and see the impact this had on him. He sat back and became a little emotional as he recollected how much this deep desire had plagued him for months leading up to his diagnosis, and how much he had enjoyed the extended time with his son.

Imagine that Jake ignored the physical, emotional, and mental signs and didn't spend time with his son. Instead, he soldiered on through the discomfort while taking painkillers to help him play golf, wakeboard, and finish his projects. The next painful message would become even more challenging than the first. This is exactly what happened.

Uncomfortable Levels of Self-Honesty

For many months Jake could feel his son needed his attention. In fact, his whole family (ecosystem) wanted more of his time. Subtle and overt messages were on display for Jake to pick up on. He just needed a painful incentive to pause his life that was running on autopilot. To take notice of not only what his family wanted but what he honestly needed.

We are an ecosystem playing around with an infinite number of other ecosystems of all shapes and sizes. It is unbelievably complex to conceptualize how it all works together. The thing is, you don't need to know how any of it works for self-healing to take place. It is like you don't need to know how the latest electric car works to enjoy the experience. It can all be so magically simple when we become aware that, in all its complexity, everything is working seamlessly together to help you get to the next part of your self-honest journey.

The more our mind opens and we see we have a bigger part to play than we thought, the more excited we get about the future because we know that not only are we playing a role in orchestrating it all, but it is all to help us. Life is designed to be effortless. It won't seem like that based on our history because in all of that time we have unknowingly been addicted to playing the blame game and practicing the art of dishonesty.

But again, life is a bullshit meter giving us feedback if we are being self-honest. Our mind, body, and environment together act as a barometer to help us take notice of the messages we receive. What makes the self-healing process more effortless is when we realize we are not only creators and not controllers, but we are receivers not foragers.

CHAPTER 11

Receivers or Foragers?

Being unaware of our addiction to playing the Blame Game means our view of the world and its possibilities is narrowed. We focus on how painful and stressful life is, and we can't see how people, events, and experiences might be helping in ways we haven't perceived yet. We are spinning around the Victim Cycle looking for new and improved ways to seek control, which keeps radical honesty at bay and slows down the healing process. While adopting a control-and-conquer strategy might help us keep our demons from the door and achieve our definition of success for a while, it isn't a permanent solution. Fear (anxiety) soon becomes a more prominent feature in our lives the more we accept and follow adrenaline-fueled sentiments like the one that popped up on my social media feed recently: "Life isn't fair! If you can't control your brain and your brain controls you, you're fucked! You have to tell your brain where you want to go and how to get there. Otherwise it is over…"

It works. But so does crack cocaine and opioids if you want to keep the demons from the door, for a while. Restrictive diets and anabolic steroids can also help you achieve success, but we know they are not sustainable solutions.

What happens as a consequence when we control our mind (brain) is that we have two opposing thoughts and beliefs running at the same time. Both in conflict. We think we have hidden, deleted, reprogrammed, rewired, or reframed our perceived negative ones, but they are always there. So as soon as we run out of energy to keep the fake positive ones going, our honest thoughts leap into action. It is why we need more intense workouts, adrenaline sports, opioids, and crack cocaine to hold back the strongest force in nature—our self-honesty.

By-Product Rather Than Force

Our control approach feels like it gives us our power back, but it actually renders us powerless. Again, it is like having a line of cocaine or a double shot of espresso for the first time. You think you can take on the world. Nothing can stop you from winning the day or week. But what about next month? Or next year? It is a fake power trip to match our fake positive mindset.

Killing everything you don't understand and that you think is getting in the way is what we have been doing for thousands of years. In that microcosm, with your blame blinkers on, this makes a lot of sense. Like the therapist who tries to "kill" the thoughts of their patient. It is a firefighting solution that might work for a while. It is not to say there isn't a place for it, but, again, is it the long-term solution?

Consider a woman who decides she wants to shed a few pounds, so she suddenly takes up tennis after decades of a sedentary lifestyle. She immediately adopts a schedule of playing an hour every other day. After a few weeks of this new regimen, her knee feels tender. She has already lost two pounds and is excited by the progress, so she decides to keep playing on her sore knee. To numb the pain, she uses ice after each game and pops a painkiller. After a few more weeks the ice and medication don't do the trick anymore, so she increases the dose to two tablets and starts wrapping her knee during the game too.

Each of these new adaptations quiets the woman's pain, makes her feel temporarily better, and allows her to continue playing tennis, lose weight, and improve her backhand. But, of course, she's not listening to what the pain is telling her. She's playing the second most popular game in the world—the waiting game. She thinks she is listening, but she is actually ignoring. The more she ignores and blames, the louder her body talks to be heard. Even when the pain escalates, she is still ignoring the message it is offering, so her blame-based fix is still the same: *How do I stop the pain?*

We all act very much like this tennis player every time we control our emotions. The self-help techniques are the equivalent of ice, painkillers, taping, orthotics, and knee wraps. By suppressing our painful feelings and replacing them with happy thoughts and motivational platitudes, we can temporarily make ourselves feel better, allowing us to play through the pain and achieve success. However, as our need to blame lessens, we naturally perceive pain and our emotions differently. Our instinct shifts from "that is negative," "this is unhelpful," or "stop holding me back" to an awareness that in the bigger picture everything is part of the honest healing process. As our perception shifts, we feel more comfortable leaning into uncomfortable feelings rather than doing all we can to run away.

Have you ever seen a film where someone is silenced by having duct tape strapped over their mouth to keep them from talking? This is what our tennis player is doing to her knee every time she blames it for doing something wrong and then wraps it up to silence its pain signals. The channel of communication is now closed. It won't be long before cortisone shots are administered, leaving only one last resort: knee surgery. Even if stem-cell therapy or some other evasive method is undertaken, it still isn't addressing her foundation that is full of blame, victimhood, and fear. It means even if the pain in her knee is silenced, other parts of her body and life will have to now become the painful mirror.

It can seem like a stretch to think our blame addiction can result in knee pain. But even if we look at this from a physiological perspective, it makes logical sense. When we are in the Victim Cycle, we are frustrated, stressed, and angry. This has an impact on our body. Even if we just focus on our neck and shoulders becoming tight, we can look at simple biomechanics.

For muscles to move, one muscle has to turn on while the other remains off. So if our upper trapezius (neck) muscle is active and scrunched up by our ears, our lower trapezius muscle is off. Meaning other muscles, like our rotator cuff complex, have to jump in to compensate to do a job they are not designed to do for long periods of time. That means all the while they are working overtime, other opposing muscles are not doing what they are meant to do. It starts a chain reaction impacting every other part of the body. It isn't long before a series of compensations lead to scar tissue forming and poor hip alignment that results in extra strain on our joints, like our knee joint. After a while it doesn't take much moving around for the knee to start talking. The question is, *Where did it all start?*

It might be easy to blame our neck muscles or the way we sit at work. But actually, our muscles didn't just randomly decide to tense up. There was something that preceded it, that told it to contract and stay contracted. It is whatever was feeding our perception that made us think something wasn't helping us. It is our blame addiction that ultimately creates our mental, emotional, and physical response (stress).

So arguably, as we start to genuinely see things as helping us discover who we honestly are, we will become less stressed. There will be fewer signals to our neck muscles to turn on and be scrunched up by our ears. Our body will then be free to do what it is designed to do—self-heal and optimally perform.

Focus on the Question Rather Than the Answer

During a client session where I was explaining this point, an image popped into my head of Sir Isaac Newton sitting under the tree where the apple bounced off his head. This is the moment he had an idea regarding gravity. Whether it's a myth or not is unimportant. For me it served its purpose, as I unexpectedly said to my client, "Humans are not foragers for answers, we are receivers." I was explaining the significance of our dreams and how they just happen. We don't get consciously involved. Control is absent. We become an open conduit to receive information, awareness, and wisdom from an unfettered place.

Receivers or Foragers?

What to call that place is a mystery. Some call it God, the Universe, or the Akashic records. Some call it our subconscious or global consciousness. I am not attached to any of those terms or concepts, as I know each comes with its own rigid connotations. I merely appreciate the infinite expanse of knowledge and guidance I have available to me while I am in this altered (blame- and control-free) state.

To get myself and my clients into this place I use *rhetorical listening*. It is a play on rhetorical questions whereby due to their very nature there is no attachment (blame) to receiving an answer. Our goal is to elicit curiosity, not pursue definitive answers. This takes practice, because we have gotten used to digging for specific answers rather than being in a state of receiving. It can feel counterintuitive that we don't need to find *core issues* for profound healing to take place. We get a buzz when we discover something that explains our perceived negative behaviors or why people treated us "badly." A sense of accomplishment arrives as we exclaim, "I've had a real shift today," but how long does the blame-hit last? How many times can we be told it was our mom, dad, sibling, or past life that messed us up before we are left exhausted wanting to give up because nothing is changing?

My point is, when it comes to honest healing, I have found the more we seek these types of answers the more it resembles a donkey following the carrot hanging inches from its nose. The anticipated reward is always just out of reach.

Psychoanalysis is another addiction we don't know we have because its repercussions go unrecognized. That is until we need psychoactive medication to counter the side effects of the monkey mind that doesn't stop (overanalysis). We swirl around again and again in the Victim Cycle looking for more core issues to explain why we are spinning out of control. It really is exhausting.

A client who had spent years in psychotherapy had a whole back catalog of stories confirming her mother and father were the reason she was in so much emotional pain and in and out of rehab. She had cycled through many therapists, and each one took a detailed account of her past, not realizing this was feeding her blame addiction.

The incessant victim-based storytelling and overanalysis confirmed my client's cognitive bias, that it was *them* that messed her up. It didn't matter how many different ways she was shown not to blame her parents, the methods being used confirmed the opposite. She learnt to push the blame deep down or transfer it onto herself. In one of our sessions, my client told me, "My father gets annoyed every time I go out in the evening." Because I didn't feed her blame addiction, and got her to look at this situation while in a state of self-honesty, it soon became evident it wasn't *every time* she went out, it was only the times she honestly didn't want to go out. Because she was blaming him for being annoying, interfering, and oppressive, she didn't see him unconsciously mirroring back her self-honesty. He stayed quiet when she honestly wanted to see friends, and unconsciously piped up when she was begrudgingly going out, because it was considered the right thing to do rather than what she really wanted to do.

A digital nomad client of mine living on a Brazilian island was trying desperately to heal from their anger and skin condition. The internet, lack of hot water, and humidity was driving them mad. The reality was, all the healing in the world wouldn't have helped them with these issues, because they honestly had enough of all the traveling. After four years on the road, they needed stability. The things that were annoying them used to be the things they loved. It is just that their priorities changed. Once they got honest and made a decision to go back to their home country for a while, they calmed down along with their rash.

When we hone our skill of receiving rather than foraging, we become open to so much more information, awareness, and guidance.

To get to this place where we can live and attain relief and freedom without the swirling, pain, and drama, we need to keep practicing a very different way of listening.

Altered State

A while ago, I started playing tennis again after a thirty-five-year hiatus. I was surprised that the movements came back to me. For the first few sessions with a coach, all was going well. I was happy with myself. Giving myself a pass for repeatedly hitting the frame or net, as I hadn't played for a long time. However, as the sessions continued, I beat myself up for my inconsistent playing. About three sessions in, I was quite pissed off with my poor performance and swung at the ball in quite an aggressive way. My shoulder started to hurt but I played through it, firmly, but unknowingly, stuck in the Victim Cycle.

I blamed my shoulder for stopping me from continuing my healthy and enjoyable pastime. I was in fear that I might have to stop.

During the next coaching session, my Achilles tendon started to hurt to the point I could hardly walk, let alone run.

This was the stimulus I needed to awaken me to the fact I was blaming myself. Instead of attempting to subdue the pain this time, I did what I had done many times before: I engaged with the pain. I went to the net and just practiced my volleys while all the time letting my shoulder and Achilles tendon know that *I am listening.* I repeated it in my head—*I am listening*—while placing my energy to any part of my body that was talking to me. I was listening in that rhetorical way where I opened the line of communication, meaning I was curious to receive any answers, which came with no attachment (blame) to their arrival.

Basically, I wasn't ignoring or blaming myself anymore. The pain lessened but was still intense enough that the session was cut short because my body said it wanted to stop. I listened, in full and honest awareness that my pain was notifying me of something that was much larger than the tennis game. In a heightened state of curiosity, with no regret or disappointment, I went back to my apartment.

As I was preparing lunch, a memory flooded in. Like a conscious dream, I saw my thirteen-year-old self smashing rackets in frustration. My shoulder and Achilles tendon started screaming at me at that precise moment. Working together, my mind and body got my attention, so I honestly listened and observed these feelings. I stopped what I was doing and stood there in front of the stove. I closed my eyes and connected with my pain and symptoms by placing 100 percent focus on them. I was in a state of curiosity. Again, as each part of my body spoke to me, I gave it the respect of my full focus and let it know I was listening.

Like a seasoned driver who knows what to do when they get in a car, I was the same when I entered this altered state.

Receivers or Foragers?

I had done enough new awareness development to know that everything that happens is helping me to connect to what I can't see. I had done enough work to know I was being helped to prepare me for the next part of my life's journey. I had a big event happening in the coming months that would take me outside my comfort zone. For that to go effortlessly, I had to become aware of where blame and feelings of victimhood and fear were playing out in my mind and body. The more I focused, the more the pain and symptoms intensified.

I realized anger was playing out under the surface and that blame was fueling my anger. I relived the memories and went deeper and deeper into the sensations. I connected, listened, felt, and observed. I let each new sensation know *I am listening* each time they spoke to me. I did the same with my thoughts. My goal was to listen in that rhetorical way rather than be attached to finding an answer or for the pain to go away. I let my unpleasant thoughts play like a tape while I gave them my full attention and respect, being very aware of how they showed up in my body.

I also knew my uncomfortable thoughts were helping me discover where I held ancestral memories in my body. Any pain I felt was just an indication of how long they had been ignored. Without these uncomfortable thoughts and sensations, my sense of victimhood would remain hidden, influencing all my perceptions, decisions, and performance. For about fifteen minutes, I had thoughts telling me: *You are shit! You are no good.* Each time a different part of my body spoke to me. The more I let the tapes play and the more I let each part of my body know the doors of communication were open, the tape ran out and the pain subsided and then disappeared. In fact, then the movie that played of me breaking my racquet became humorous when it was no longer accompanied by self-blame. The memory changed as a by-product of the listening and healing, not because I forced it to change or used any technique to change it into what I thought was a positive alternative.

At our next practice session, my coach couldn't understand how I had gotten so much better. He commented that I looked so much more relaxed. All I had done was engage with the honest healing process and rhetorically listen to my feelings rather than pushing them away (blaming and ignoring them).

Like the example of driving a car. Initially driving on the road feels like a nightmare. So much stress. But later you wonder what all the worry and stress was about. We get in the car and it is effortless. Self-healing is also designed to be simple and effortless. That doesn't mean it will be easy. But that doesn't mean it will be hard or difficult either.

It Can't Be That Simple!

A client once asked me at the end of our session, "Oh, can you quickly help with any advice on my nosebleeds? I have had them every day for the last seven years." I simply asked her, "Do you think your nose is doing something wrong?" "Yes," was the quick response. I asked if she would say the same if her body was giving her signs to drink more water? "Of course not," she said. I continued, "Is it fair to say that you don't know what your nose is telling you but it is telling you something that is helpful?"

After she agreed, I reminded her that she was blaming her nose for doing something wrong, and then because she had accepted it as part of her life, she was ignoring it. Hoping it would go away in time.

I told her the story of my tennis lessons and asked her to open the door of communication with her nose. That's it. Nothing else. A month later she emailed me in a state of confusion. Her nose stopped bleeding the day after our session and hadn't bled since.

The confusion came from the fact she didn't get an answer to what was causing the bleeding, or how it was helping her. So as much as she liked the result, she couldn't fully enjoy it because she was still attached to finding the answer. I understood, because she wanted to know what she'd done so she could do the same if it happened again. She was in the *I need to learn from my mistakes* mindset. The funny thing is, she did know the answer and she did know what to do if anything like this happened again: honestly listen. But it felt too simple even though it had worked for this and other issues in her life.

I now enjoy noticing how I change while not knowing why. If I receive answers, great; if I don't, great. This for me is an important part of experiencing true freedom. It is also why I go into the honest healing space when I am feeling great. I'm not waiting until my mind, body, or life is screaming at me for attention—I get a massage before I *need* a massage. The *prevention rather than cure* mentality is something that has significantly helped me enjoy the effortlessness that I experience. This was highlighted to me many moons ago when a client sent me a message saying, "I know I haven't been in touch for a while but I have been waiting for something to happen so I don't waste my session with you."

The point is, going into the honest healing and listening space when you are relaxed, happy, and full of energy is the equivalent of doing physical exercise when you are in the same mindset. It's going to be a more enjoyable experience. If you are in a lot of physical or emotional pain, you might find it harder to listen in a rhetorical way. You will just want to stop the pain. This is why I don't discourage my clients from using coping mechanisms. Sometimes we have to do whatever we have to do to quell the emotional and physical pain. However, I do have a caveat. Once the pain has subsided, this is the time to do the self-healing work outlined in this book. It sounds counterintuitive to evoke painful memories when we are feeling in a "good place," but staying in the artificially induced comfort isn't going to last anyway, regardless of how powerful the sedative was. This is a great window of opportunity to self-reflect while in a curious state of mind.

We have all been accumulating mountains of evidence throughout our entire lives proving that the world is full of hardship, struggle, pain, and suffering. We think extreme pain is normal and others are out to get us. But this is because all the help we have available is feeding our addiction to blame. Many clients can feel overwhelmed on the blame-recovery journey as it opens floodgates they didn't know they had been erecting. It can feel like an existential crisis as we shed our victim identity—the very skin we have become so accustomed to.

As we recover from our blame addiction, it can leave us raw as we gain access to everything we have been trying to ignore. We have so many avenues (books, seminars, podcasts, courses, videos, gurus, films) to get our blame fix without knowing it. They come with the same victim/hero story and control-and-conquer solutions. It leads us to think that we have so much stuff to work through, which in itself can result in us thinking, "What's the point?" when in fact, honest healing acts like a domino effect. You are working with your very foundation. When that changes, so many of our victim stories effortlessly fall away. We really are not as f'ed up as we think we are.

All our victim stories are predicated on the notion there is an ideal way to behave. It instills the fear that we have, are, or will do something wrong. The truth of the matter is, if we followed all the expert advice around nutrition we wouldn't eat or drink anything. The same is true of parenting. Yes parents, you are doing it wrong! Some expert, somewhere in the world, is telling you what the right way is, and you ain't doing it. And even if you are parenting and living the ideal way, does this guarantee you will get the results that are promised to you? Based on all the different interpretations in the world, we are always doing something "wrong." It is why in my coaching sessions I am not telling people what to do. I want them to honestly heal so their decisions take them towards optimal health and joy, rather than an extreme experience to find out where they are blaming. This attachment to fictitious ideals smothers our innate wisdom—the part of us that understands everyone and everything is here to help us find out who we honestly are and never to hold us back.

As I gained more new awareness around my blame addiction and where I was unknowingly feeding it, the rhetorical listening space became more enjoyable. To help me with this, I had to understand the most misunderstood emotion we have—fear—while becoming aware of how powerful why-based questions are—but not in the way you may think.

CHAPTER 12

Fear—Friend or Foe?

It might not seem like it, but asking why-based questions is a contributing factor to why fear is such a common companion in our life.

Why am I so angry? Why am I so anxious? Why is my thyroid not working properly? Why? Why? Why? Is it me, or does why just lead to more whys? And the more I don't know why, the more fearful I get.

After thousands of years marauding through life perfecting our ability to control and conquer anything we think is standing in our way—including our mind, body, and soul—we have taught ourselves to be expert blamers and masterful victims. It means we haven't noticed that it is only when we are blaming and being a victim that we think something is bad, negative, wrong, a mistake, or a failure. And it is only when we think in this dualistic and dichotomous way that we are angry, fearful (anxious), stressed, and ill.

When we aren't suppressing our fear and anger, we're overwhelmed and seething with it. Many of us find ourselves regularly pissed off about anything and everything. We're livid at the terrible politician, president, or prime minister. We're furious at our partner for playing video games instead of watching a film with us. We even go off the deep end when a car doesn't react like a Formula One race car as the traffic light turns green.

It can be confusing because we are getting more angry with the small things in our life. We might even pride ourselves on being calm when under fire, but as soon as someone doesn't say sorry or thank you when you think they should, you are left in disbelief at what comes out of your mouth. Our ability to control our anger is becoming harder, and it is making us afraid of what we are capable of if the beast is let loose.

When we're in the throes of anger we naturally believe it is someone else's fault. We have been wronged, damn it. Blinded by the red mist, we don't appreciate how anger is an indicator that we are in the later stages of our blame addiction, and the longer we ignore this, the more it shows up as chronic inflammation in our body. For example, many of the same people with anger issues have diagnoses and labels that suggest they have malfunctioning thyroids. Not realizing their thyroids aren't acting up, they are simply responding perfectly to what the other glands in their body are doing. When controlling it with medication no longer works, the final solution is to surgically remove it.

However, when you use your blame-dar, you can see this is the second option and final phase of your blame addiction. After putting up with (controlling/accepting) something you have been blaming for a long time, you cut it out of your life. It stands to reason, if the anger wasn't there your body would function differently. We know this logically, which is why we are told to reduce our stress. But all the ways we have been trying to reduce our stress and control our anger (and fear) have been blame-based.

Even when we venture into our past to see if healing our anger can be found there, we go in looking for what went wrong and then try to find out why it happened. All in the hope that if we can understand it, we will fix it and find some relief. What ends up happening is we keep getting dopamine highs from working stuff out, not realizing it is keeping us in the Victim Cycle, which amplifies our fear and anger.

The reality is we might not be able to change the experience we had, but our perception of it can change when we address what is in our foundation. To help with this, we must recognize the victim-inducing power of questions, starting with "Why?"

Why Me!

"Why?" is one of the most important words in the English Language. In his famous TED Talk, "How great leaders inspire action" and his bestselling book *Start With Why*, Simon Sinek advised us to find our purpose and reason for existing and place it front and center so others will also care as much as we do. He explained that, "People don't buy WHAT you do; they buy WHY you do it." Sinek's talks and books are popular because his message is valid. When it comes to business, asking why can create connection with the target audience. However, when it comes to honest healing, happiness, and transformation, "why" can create something very different.

Why we do what we do is the elusive question philosophers and historians have pondered for thousands of years. Modern-day psychologists spend their careers attempting to unravel the mysteries of the human mind. Like a prospector looking for nuggets of gold in the middle of a mountain stream, they search our subconscious mind for pieces of information that will bring great rewards. However, as logical as it seems, once again this approach feeds our addiction to blame.

Venturing down these rabbit holes is satisfying because it provides the intellectual dopamine hit we didn't know we needed. Before long we are like a kid mimicking a cowboy gunslinger, pumping our blame fingers back and forth hitting anything we think is standing in our way (including ourselves). Psychoanalyzing our past looking for core issues as to why we did what we did, or why others did what they did, is like a new diet reaching the market that had a too-good-to-be-true promise of significant weight loss by consuming a lot of refined sugar. Any sugar addict will jump at the opportunity to see if it works. And even when they are getting fatter, they have bought into the propaganda and keep going. Surely next week they will start getting results. Finally, they become obese and blame the person who invented the diet. Similarly, blame addicts love the idea of modern medical, psychological, spiritual, and new age approaches to healing because these ideologies all feed our unknown addiction.

In the end, all our why-based questions are variations of the same theme: "Why me?" "Why do these bad things keep happening to me?" We are telling ourselves a victim story without realizing it. This leads to mental, emotional, and physical exhaustion, which then gets diagnosed as "depression" or some other label that can be medicated. I can sound skeptical of this approach because I am. I know the control-and-conquer approach helped many people, including myself, but it is perpetuated as the only answer. And even the results we get are short-term.

Before I realized the impact of why-based questions for honest healing, I kept coming up with new ones: Why did I say that? Why didn't I just tell them no? Why is this happening to me? Why did they act in that way? Why are you shouting at me? Why did you take advantage of my good nature? Why am I holding myself back? Why are you sabotaging me from reaching my goals? Why, why, why just led to more whys. These questions all led back to the same idea: Why me! I am a good person; I don't deserve this type of negative treatment! Life is unfair! Life is against me! It is an exhausting line of questioning and results in us feeling "stuck" in life.

As always, "why" isn't the enemy. I use it, but my relationship with it has changed.

To listen in a way that facilitates honest healing, we need new awareness. Finding out why we or others do what we do is vital if we want to find out how to manipulate someone into buying something. Investigating the human psyche is of paramount importance to any magician, hypnotist, or mentalist if they want to continue to wow their audience. Even a forensic scientist or detective needs to know behavioral science to be able to capture their suspect. In this respect, being curious about our psychological makeup is helpful, entertaining, and fascinating.

"Why" is also essential when we are building a machine or computer. We need to know why the feeder keeps jamming in our printer. We must investigate why the code keeps kicking off that error message. We have to determine why the grid is always overloading. For mechanics and engineers, asking why is helpful.

Contrary to popular belief, the human being is not a machine and it doesn't resemble a computer. These archaic and antiquated analogies lead us to think we need to be manipulated and fixed when we do something we don't understand or perceive as bad, negative, wrong, a mistake, or a failure.

Asking why has a tendency to keep us feeling like we're walking through a labyrinth looking for a diamond in the rough. It creates attachment to finding answers based on rigid ideals around what is considered a good or bad result. The goal is to wean ourselves off the dopamine hit that comes when we gain some intellectual realization that makes us feel like we're winning the Blame Game. Finding a belief that we think is sabotaging us, shooting us in the foot, or blocking us from happiness and financial abundance can feel great. But the blame remains. So even if our financial situation changes due to renewed energy that comes with the dopamine high, the blame has to reveal itself somewhere else in our life. This is why drama seems to keep following us and why our "good times don't last long."

The main reason it becomes exhausting to seek answers and follow why-based enquiry when it comes to honest healing is because of where we place the emphasis. When we ask why we are not actually curious about learning about ourselves or accessing our self-honesty, we just want the pain to stop. More victim-based questions follow: Why am I doing these *bad* things to *sabotage* myself? Why do I keep attracting the same *negative* people and experiences into my life? Why do I keep repeating the same *bad* patterns that are holding me back? Why do I keep doing everything *wrong* and making *mistakes*? Why is my inner saboteur making me a *failure*? The list is endless. And any answer we get will confirm we are a victim whether we are aware of it or not.

Once the exhaustion reaches a certain point, we default to a common mantra: Why do we have to keep experiencing so much pain? Why does life seem so hard? Again, it is not that "why" is the enemy. It is that it has become synonymous with "Why me!" It is the reason I very rarely engage with this line of questioning. The second reason is that there is a simple and universal answer to explain all my victim-based stories and any why-based questions. Regardless of the circumstances, the answer to why is: because you are blaming yourself or others for doing something they shouldn't have. Your ideal didn't come to fruition. Classing something as wrong while having incomplete information, awareness, and wisdom is the foundation of any painful emotion, symptom, pain, addiction, or experience.

This blame-infused foundation has been with us since birth. This is why we need to co-create a stimulus big enough to break through all our denial and control-and-conquer strategies to access the self-honesty that is underneath. It is easy to call something wrong at the extreme end of the scale, but if it was addressed at the start, then it would never reach a point where it would be regarded as wrong.

Why do we have to experience extreme levels of pain? Because we have different degrees of ignorance and denial to make our way through. So anytime you might ask yourself a why-based question—you do know why. The answer is the same. It is the reason we co-create everything in our lives: to help us find out where we are blaming and where it is stored in our body so we can exit the Victim Cycle. All so we can get self-honest and heal to finally get to know who we honestly are. And then create a life based on the honest us.

When we are fearful or angry, it's an indicator that blame is in the air and we are being asked to listen to reach new levels of self-honesty.

Fear—Friend or Foe?

Fear is one of the most misunderstood emotions we have. Many successful athletes, actors, leaders, doctors, and parents have expressed the importance of fear, whether it drives their motivation to train, learn lines, hit sales targets, encourage patients to take medication, or get children to brush their teeth.

At the same time, fear is seen as the main reason we hold ourselves back in life. It is fear's fault that we don't step outside our comfort zone and follow our dreams. So is fear helping us or holding us back?

When facilitating a group in Argentina, participants looked at me as if I was crazy. I had just suggested that fear is our friend and is always helping and guiding us. And in fact, it never holds us back from anything. Some participants told me that something had obviously been lost in translation. Many of them assured me that fear is most definitely not their friend. It is something to beat, overcome, and control before it does the same to you. Many successful people have said the same. Your fearful thoughts are a virus that need to be controlled, beaten into submission, and overcome.

This age-old control-and-conquer approach to fear is unquestionable. It has stood the test of time, so why try to fix what isn't broken? Because this approach isn't conducive to long-term and honest healing. It creates a paradigm where fear is the bully and we are its victim. It taps into our blame-based need to get revenge on the thing (or person) we think is hurting and holding us back.

The masculine, stoic control approach to life fears anything it doesn't understand. It is why we fear fear. We treat fear like fighting with a lifeguard who is saving us from drowning. We think being flipped on our back and having an arm thrust around our chest or neck is a bad thing. Thinking they are making the situation worse, we panic and fight back. However, once we are lying on the beach alive and relieved, it all makes sense. The point is that our fearful experiences can be much less physically and mentally stressful if we become aware that fear is always helping us.

The reality is: fear is not the problem, enemy, or bully. What needs our attention is whatever is feeding our perception making us fear a particular outcome. Once our foundation changes, once blame and victimhood start to vacate, fear follows automatically.

To help change our relationship with fear, we need to once again ignite our curiosity—the unsung hero that continues to help us on the road to honest healing where profound freedom and happiness is to be found.

Curiosity results in wonder. Wonder is the amazement at something beautiful, remarkable, or unfamiliar. This is the essence of what life is about. It is what provides the incentive and fuel for adventure. It helps us find out who we honestly are. Without curiosity, our passion for living dwindles like a candle running out of wax, leaving no energy to find or keep our purpose alight. And arguably, without purpose there is no will or desire to learn anything new, step outside our comfort zone, or question our rigid beliefs. As much as establishing boundaries and *sticking with what you know* can maintain a sense of calm and control, it is an illusion, as nothing can hold back our self-honesty that is constantly pushing through to help us find meaning and purpose.

In a world where the mainstream approach to teaching children is through rote learning and memorizing facts and figures, curiosity is often left on the bench waiting for its moment to shine. All the time I was jumping from one job to the next in London's rat race, my candle was running out and my mind closed down to conserve energy. It wasn't until my unceremonious departure from my last office job that my curiosity sprung to life after a long hiatus. Learning to be a personal trainer was the catalyst for me to wonder at life again. To take a peek over the ditch of despair I was in, to notice just enough beauty and possibility to awaken my need to venture into the unfamiliar.

I didn't realize it at the time, but the antidote to fear is an honestly open mind, not the fake one we promote to get people to like us. Fear is present when we have our blame blinkers on. It is like hearing a noise in the middle of the night. Because we don't have all the information, we can only see bad, negative, and wrong scenarios play out. When the light goes on and we see the cat wandering around, the fear naturally disappears.

In the same way, how would you feel if your partner came home and told you that a stranger had rubbed their hands all over their body for an hour? You may not be impressed and fear your relationship has ended. That is, until your partner tells you that they had a massage. At which point, with one piece of information your perception completely shifts and suddenly the blame has gone, the victimhood is no longer present, and no fear or anger is to be seen.

Our rising blame and fear have resulted in a movement to erect literal and virtual boundaries all around ourselves to make sure we are not emotionally and physically hurt. It is a sign we are in the Victim Cycle and putting up walls of blame and denial. And as I have mentioned many times, the longer we are in the cycle, the more extreme the pain needs to be to help us notice that we are in it so we can start the process of exiting.

While in this fearful state we forget that the only person who can emotionally hurt us is us. It has nothing to do with what the other person said or did. Based on our known or hidden agenda, we just interpreted (blamed) whatever they did as wrong. Simply put, fear effortlessly leaves us as we recover from our blame addiction. But our ability to sense danger remains. By focusing on eradicating fear from our lives, we have inadvertently been feeding it. It is why fear is so rampant. It gets a little more complicated in our modern world because it is now known by a different name.

Fear has had a makeover that has created more blame and postponed our ability to honestly heal.

My Anxiety Is Holding Me Back

While growing up, I'd never heard of anxiety, but now it's mentioned in most of my client sessions. Some tell me it is a mild concern, while others complain their anxiety is so debilitating that it's a daily struggle to combat and overcome the nervousness, uneasiness, and apprehension they experience. Either way, my response is the same: when we keep it simple, anxiety is just another word for fear.

When someone is in a state of extreme fear, such as being confronted by their phobia of public speaking, they can behave in the same way as someone who is said to be having a panic attack. I make sure my clients know that fear has effectively been repackaged as anxiety. This way it can be classified as a disorder, meaning it can be medicated and treated differently than someone who simply says they are scared or worried. Credit where credit is due—rebranding fear so new products and services can be offered is a genius business and marketing ploy. Especially when fear levels around the globe are at an all-time high.

If we treat them as one and the same and apply what we have covered so far in the book, it is clear that the reason we are afraid is because we think we are being held back and something bad, negative, wrong, a mistake, or a failure is going to happen. When we start to realize that everyone and everything is helping us uncover who we honestly are and never holding us back, anxiety no longer has any fuel to keep it going.

A musician client of mine who told me she suffered a lot from anxiety found much relief once she no longer accepted the fallacy around her various labels like "generalized anxiety disorder (GAD)," "panic disorder," and "social anxiety disorder." After seeing fear and anxiety as the same thing and as a friend not foe, she learned to give all her symptoms what they wanted—100 percent of her focus, rather than being blamed, ignored, and told to shut up with medication or coping mechanisms. The more she practiced honestly listening, the more she realized just how much it had been helping and guiding her.

For example, while my client was on tour, there had been times she didn't really want to party with the band members and crew, so she had used her anxiety as an excuse to bail out. No one questioned this, as everyone had been informed that she may have panic attacks if she didn't get enough rest. In essence, she had crafted a guilt-free reason to get out of any situation she didn't want to be in. She admitted that there were times she consciously knew she was doing this, and other times she was completely unaware this was happening.

As she opened one door into her self-honesty, others opened. She realized she used her label of anxiety disorder to get out of family gatherings or seeing friends that she had been blaming for draining her energy and causing her "anxiety." She felt so much lighter in mind and body after accessing this level of self-honesty, but we reached a sticking point. What about when she *really* wanted to do something and fear stopped her? She asked me, "Why would I have this bad reaction when something good or exciting is happening?"

Instead of giving her the answer, I asked my client to go home and spend time in the honest listening space. I reminded her to rhetorically listen and observe her thoughts and physical sensations. While she was in this space, I said, "You think fear is stopping you from doing what you wholeheartedly want to do. Instead of focusing there, ponder the idea that just because your conscious plan didn't happen that maybe your more influential unconscious [self-honest] plan did." It was a way of encouraging her to reconsider labeling her reactions as bad or wrong, but rather just as information for her to be curious about exploring.

She told me that sitting in silence while accessing times she had a panic attack felt very uncomfortable. However, she stayed with the process and gradually connections started to show up. As much as we don't need to receive answers for emotional and physical healing to take place, eureka moments can happen. For my client, it took a number of listening sessions over a week for a big realization to arrive. And when it did, all her chronic back pain disappeared.

She told me about a time she was supposed to go to an important rehearsal but instead became so fearful (anxious) that she couldn't leave the house. With renewed self-honesty, she could see her overriding desire: her priority was to spend time with her husband, whom she hadn't seen for a long time. It was that night they conceived their first child.

This was one of those weird and wonderful moments that can't be explained or enjoyed while we are whirling around in the Victim Cycle looking for labels and disorders to blame our experiences and feelings on.

Calling something bad or negative and deferring responsibility is easy. Beating ourselves up for doing wrong is easy. Questioning what we have been told is true, self-reflecting, getting self-honest, and exploring other possible versions of our victim stories can also be easy. Like any other skill we learn, it takes specific practice for it to become effortless.

As soon as we see something as the enemy or holding us back, it is an indication we are in the Victim Cycle. In contrast, when we start to explore all the possible ways we contributed and how we have been or are being helped, it is a sign we are exiting. This can sound like I am advocating for a positive mental attitude, but there are a few significant differences. When we are looking for positives we are anchoring that there was a negative and we are being held back. Developing a Positive Mental Attitude (PMA) has a fake-it-till-you-make-it mentality behind it. It teaches us to be dishonest with ourselves and others. It also promotes using control to survive the experience that is thought to have gone sideways. While in this mindset, we might conclude, "It is what it is. There is no point in complaining, we should just move on." Like all control measures, it works. But like all control measures, it isn't sustainable.

It can feel empowering to brush off our honest feelings of being angry or disappointed with, "Everything happens for a reason." We might even be able to push enough painful memories under the rug with, "My past made me who I am today." This might work if you have your health, a roof over your head, and food in the fridge. But what if you don't have these basic essentials? Is saying your so-called bad experiences made you who you are today going to make you feel empowered, or is it going to be the perfect mantra to beat yourself up with? Seeing the cup as half full and looking for the silver lining works for a while. But it doesn't fundamentally alter what is in our foundation. Each fake positive platitude is just another layer we put between us and our self-honesty.

The goal is to fundamentally heal from our blame addiction so as a by-product the foundation of our mindset changes. This way we no longer see a *negative* to turn into a positive. We recognize that experiences don't get worse, they get incrementally more extreme. The longer we play the waiting game, the message (mirror) has to get as big, loud, and painful as it needs to in order to shake us out of our denial or ignorance. This way we can see where our blame addiction is being fed, so it can be listened to and healed.

It is easy to get caught up with blaming others for being evil or for getting fixated on their perceived intention to hurt or sabotage you. Many clients believe their mothers-in-law have one mission in life—to make sure they are miserable. They throw around accusations that they are trying all they can to end the marriage with their son. This is the easy victim route. Self-reflecting on your self-honesty, asking whether you are wholeheartedly happy in your marriage, or if some other deep truth is pushing through, might be a harder pill to swallow. But until you spend time with your self-honesty (and body) listening, the mother-in-law's behavior will have to keep getting more extreme. Not because they are getting more evil, but because they have to play their part, even if it is unconsciously, to help you get deeply self-honest with yourself.

As one client confirmed to me after doing the mirror list on Cruella (her mother-in-law's nickname), she felt incredibly uncomfortable as she recognized she had similar tendencies and characteristics. What was even more shocking was her admittance to herself that she was a lesbian. She had known it before she got married but passed it off as a phase. Her so-called evil mother-in-law was unconsciously pushing incrementally harder and harder to get my client to be honest with herself about many things.

To help us really grasp why our situations get ever more extreme, we have to see how everything is working symbiotically to help the whole.

Nothing Is Random

Nature constantly demonstrates that when blame-filled humans are not present, it has a beautiful ebb and flow. All that happens is wonderfully orchestrated in the way it works together. There is no blame-based interpretation to interfere with its perfection, and it flourishes. When we look to control any part of the ecosystem, we find ourselves in a battle of wills, and it incrementally decays.

As I mentioned before, nature is always looking to flourish—it doesn't understand survival. It isn't looking to get by, even if that is what it looks like. Since we are part of nature, we have the same potential. It is only our addiction to playing the Blame Game and all the blame-based perceptions, concepts, and theories that emerge that makes us feel separated from ourselves, others, and nature.

I suppose the questions at this point are: Do you believe everything is symbiotically connected to everything else in some way? Or do you think randomness exists in nature?

There are some key people of influence that think we just might all be interconnected:

> *"Learn how to see. Realize that everything connects to everything else."*
> —LEONARDO DA VINCI

> *"When we try to pick out anything by itself, we find it hitched to everything else in the Universe."*
> —JOHN MUIR

> *"Whatever affects one directly, affects all indirectly."*
> —MARTIN LUTHER KING JR.

"I'll tell you what hermits realize. If you go off into a far, far forest and get very quiet, you'll come to understand that you're connected with everything."

—ALAN WATTS

Of course, I have chosen people to back up my cognitive bias. We could just accept that everything is random and chaotic. I've been there and done that, and it just led to more victim stories. When we have our blame blinkers on, life seems like it is full of random, chaotic, and coincidental moments.

It is like when people moved from their first black-and-white TV to a color one. The excitement was tangible as they saw in a way that was previously thought impossible. The same is true for my clients, who only see in rigid right-and-wrong ways based on their blame-infused perspectives. As they gain access to their self-honesty, the color of possibility reveals itself.

Believing that random events happen gives us wiggle room to be a victim. It makes us believe we need more control or acceptance. However, more information, awareness, and wisdom are always available. No event, experience, or decision is made in isolation. There is always a whole theater production going on behind the scenes.

All the while we dichotomize our experiences into rigidly helpful or unhelpful, we are in the blaming, shaming, and ignoring mindset. We see it play out with interviewers who have a specific agenda. They push the guest for a yes or no answer. The need for a dichotomous answer is a powerful tool in a propagandist arsenal, as it negates any nuance the interviewee is attempting to explain. In any situation there is more at play. For example, when a friend forgets to set their alarm leaving you standing at your front door looking at your watch when you should be on your way to the airport, you get angry and upset and make fear- and panic-driven decisions. The red mist only allows you to see bad, negative, and wrong scenarios. But could more be playing out?

It goes unrecognized that we were sending subliminal messages to our friend to not pick us up. When they asked us if we were looking forward to the trip, we nonchalantly shrugged our shoulders, scrunched up our face, and in a monotone way said, "Yeah, well, yeah-no…it should be fun."

Magicians, mentalists, and marketeers have perfected subliminal messaging and neuromarketing techniques. The 2015 film *Focus* with Will Smith perfectly illustrates what is possible. Communication is often invisible or imperceptible. Nikola Tesla said, "If you want to know the secrets of the universe, see it in terms of energy, frequency, and vibration." An ecosystem is a set of dynamically connected elements. If you do something to any one of them, the others are also affected. Families, teams, departments, and organizations are dynamically connected too. Nothing happens randomly or in isolation because there is energy, frequency, and vibration always present. They all carry information, like invisible pheromones helping a line of ants navigate the jungle floor.

A few years ago, a client came to see me about her paralyzing fear of public speaking. She had been asked to give a pivotal presentation to over a hundred company executives that could solidify a relationship with one of her main clients. She was terrified. She didn't want to be the reason her company lost the client. On her way to the presentation, her taxi hit another car. She was shaken and had minor physical injuries. This was a defining moment. She was at the proverbial (and physical) crossroads. She had the perfect guilt-free excuse to skip her presentation. But she'd been working with me for some time and, instead of blaming anyone for the predicament, she listened. She sat with herself long enough to really listen and be self-honest.

And what did she hear? All of a sudden, she had an overwhelming urge to get to the conference. She jumped out of the taxi, ran to the nearest subway station, and ran all the way to the venue just in time to step out on stage. She realized she wanted to give a great presentation more than she wanted to avoid public speaking. But there was something else playing out that she was completely unaware of, and it was going to help her in unimaginable ways.

The two scariest moments for someone giving a speech are waiting to go on stage and saying the first words. Is it random that the car crash occupied all her attention and filled her full of stress-relieving adrenaline? Is it a coincidence that by the time she reached the venue she felt no fear and she now had an honest, dramatic, and captivating story to open her speech with?

Maybe!

But maybe not...

Many ancient philosophers and wisdom keepers spent extended periods of time in nature. I did the same as I traveled around the globe and experienced all different types of ecosystems. And when you sit and observe, something happens to you. Something very unexpected. You start to see how it is all beautifully orchestrated. How everything works symbiotically together. Yes, you can read about this, or watch the latest David

Attenborough documentary, which are all recommended. But nothing compares to sitting and observing nature while simply listening. Not trying to understand it. Not trying to work anything out. Just connecting and listening. You start to realize that maybe, just maybe, life is all beautifully orchestrated and a blessing in disguise.

A Blessing in Disguise

Many people in today's world adopt the rational view that our existence is made up of random and chaotic events. However, it often seems that after we deem something as random, someone writes a scientific paper detailing a new discovery that shows it was no such thing. In fact, this is the purpose of science—to make connections where there seemed to be none before. Things only seem random when we don't understand them. After we gain wisdom and widen our perception, we see patterns behind things that appeared coincidental.

As Agent K said in the film *Men in Black*, "Fifteen hundred years ago everybody knew the Earth was the center of the universe. Five hundred years ago, everybody knew the Earth was flat, and fifteen minutes ago, you knew that humans were alone on this planet. Imagine what you'll know tomorrow." What will we know if CERN, the European Organization for Nuclear Research, discovers dark matter? What will happen if we accelerate our bioengineering ability from enabling rats to grow new limbs to humans? Isn't it always just a matter of time before we realize anything is possible in time and everything is connected?

Believing events are random complicates the honest healing process. This belief shuts down our curiosity. It is easy to just say "that is random" or "unfair" when we don't fully understand something. Accidents, sickness, bad luck, malice, and natural disasters are all easy to write off as unfortunate parts of being human. All these events are considered random and "out of our control." But is this actually the case?

With more information, awareness, and wisdom, things we once thought were random in fact make a lot of sense. Sometimes we even hear ourselves say, "That was a blessing in disguise."

After being different than other girls due to developing large breasts at a young age, Elisha became anxious and depressed due to the attention she received. In her early twenties she developed lumps on her breasts. This news was obviously heart-wrenching for friends and family. But Elisha secretly saw her diagnosis differently.

The decision was made to have the lumps surgically removed. It was also decided as a preventative measure, Elisha would have a breast reduction. Before I had a chance to offer my thoughts around this not being random, she told me the realization she had at the time of the news. She said, "I saw the lumps as a blessing in disguise."

Elisha knew it wasn't random, but she kept her thoughts to herself because she didn't want to be seen as crazy.

After I offered this perspective to a different client, she found it confusing. "But Denis," she began, "it is a fact, there are bad things in the world. There are human rights issues, genocide, famine, criminals killing people, pharmaceutical companies marketing their addictive drugs, pedophiles molesting children, and governments passing policies that negatively impact others. How are the people on the receiving end of these abuses not innocent victims?" I agreed with her in one sense: the list of all the places we could lay fault for the things we label as bad, negative, and wrong is essentially endless.

"Has our victimizing the victim approach helped," I asked, "to reduce or stop these painful situations from happening? Has seeing certain events as random helped us in any way to heal and change as individuals or as a species?"

She shook her head. "What can we do?" she asked. "What would put an end to the world's atrocities?"

"You're already doing it," I told her. "You're already on the journey to exit the Victim Cycle. As you do, you will help the planet and all its inhabitants heal in the most profound way possible."

It can sound too simple, but when we exit the Victim Cycle and heal, it has a ripple effect. It becomes infectious for others to want to do the same. The less blame there is in any ecosystem, the more it harmonizes. There is no sense of victimhood, fear, or anger to fuel the desire for revenge, abuse, dominance, or control.

Self-healing is neither easy nor hard, but it is simple. We just have to start a new cycle to exit the one we have been in for thousands of years.

CHAPTER 13

Self-Healing Cycle

At some point while working with clients, I let them know they don't have to live the way I do. I am not shy to say I have been obsessed with living a life where there is no wiggle room to be a victim for nearly fifteen years. With that said, I am still open to finding where I am unknowingly feeding my addiction to blame. It can show up like it did when I was playing tennis years ago. It might happen while taking this book on tour. Either way, I am all in as I personally see and enjoy the benefits of living this victimless way.

Not everyone wants to be a world-class basketball player. They enjoy shooting hoops on the weekend. It is enough to keep connected with friends and at the fitness level they are happy with. The same is true here. Applying what you have learnt so far and entering the self-healing space now and then will bring many welcome emotional, mental, and physical benefits. You don't have to dive in with two feet and remain there like me. I say this because you could end the book here. And if you regularly reread the chapters above, your life would fundamentally change in a way you would very much enjoy. The rest of the book is for people that want to go the extra mile and reach another level of freedom and confidence. To experience this, you will be venturing into the possibility that we really do contribute to *everything* that happens in our life as an individual and as a species.

Being dedicated as much as I have been to see what life looks like when blame, victimhood, fear, and control are no longer my main drivers has been uncomfortable at times. I had to recognize that I played a role in co-creating everything that happens in my life. This was relatively easy to do when it came to interpersonal situations like arguments, breakups, and missing flights. But in other situations, it took new awareness and more honest listening to see my contribution.

What If I Really Am a Victim?

We have plenty of crimes where we specifically use the word "victim" to describe one of the parties. For instance, a kid whose parent physically beats her is said to be a victim of child abuse. Similarly, we often hear about rape victims, murder victims, and victims of identity theft. Further, there are victims of natural disasters.

Surely the victim of identity theft can't be held as partly responsible. A rape victim cannot be said to have co-created abuse along with the rapist, right? And the victims of the latest hurricane certainly couldn't have co-created that natural disaster, could they have? Surely this is a classic case of "victim blaming."

My goal is not to assign blame or victimhood anywhere. I want to help people exit their victim mindset so we all co-create a very different world to the one we have gotten used to. The by-product of the blame-recovery process is more harmony, empathy, joy, and confidence. Abuse, conflict, and addiction of any type can't exist in this environment.

If someone told you it was the fifth time their identity had been stolen, would you inquire how they might be contributing to this? What about if three of your last relationships cheated on you? Would you consider looking at yourself to see where you might be playing your part? If someone's house had been destroyed by a hurricane, you might consider them an innocent victim. As a one-off this might be an easy conclusion. But what if they built or bought another house in the same place and the same thing happened—would you call them an innocent victim then? Did they have anything to contribute to that experience? Can they claim to be an innocent victim every time their house is destroyed?

What if someone was standing on the sidewalk and a drunk driver mounted the curb and hit them? Can the pedestrian take any responsibility for their part in this experience? On the surface it is an easy answer—no! But what if you found out the person on the curb was distracted by playing a game on their phone at the time of impact? Many people I have offered this scenario to tell me it doesn't matter—they are an innocent victim because the driver was drunk. What they did was wrong. That is why I use a drunk driver—it adds moral indignation to the scenario. I then ask, "If you found a suicide note on the person who got hit, could this be considered their contribution to the experience?"

The issue is that when something so extreme happens, we jump to our black-and-white thinking. Our mind shuts down and we seek justice or revenge. This is why propaganda works so well when the target audience is in a state of fear, uncertainty, and doubt (victim mindset). With my scenario, we get hooked on the fact the driver is drunk. We then assume the pedestrian was doing nothing "wrong" and just minding their own business and this "bad" thing happened to them. But that is like saying we don't have to be observant and aware of our surroundings when we are in the apparent safe zone of the sidewalk.

The reality is, if the pedestrian was on their way to kill themselves, then they may have seen the car but didn't move. We don't have to go to this extreme possibility. The person could see this as an opportunity to get an insurance payout. There are lots of comical displays on social media where people are jumping in front of cars acting like they have been hurt. It is not about justifying the drunk driver. It is to illustrate that with more information, awareness, and wisdom, more light is shed on the situation opening us to other possibilities.

The people who commit the horrendous acts of abuse happening all around the world are in the extreme stage of their blame addiction. They have become separated from themselves and others. They seek out vulnerable people, those who are deeply in the Victim Cycle. I understand what Dr. Brené Brown was saying in her popular TedTalk, "The Power of Vulnerability," but if you look at the definition a very different picture is painted. The goal is to get us to be open and share our feelings, but vulnerability actually means "open to attack." Susceptible to physical and emotional harm and easily hurt. This is encouraging someone to remain in their victim mindset. It can initially feel good to be in this state as it is feeding our blame addiction, because we will inevitably get upset as we accuse someone of attacking us or taking advantage of our vulnerability. By blaming them we don't realize our contribution to the experience. We opened ourselves to attack and got attacked.

All the while we are being encouraged to be a victim (knowingly or unknowingly), it means we are not being self-honest. However, when we are in this honest self-reflective state, we are able to be open and comfortable sharing our feelings and thoughts. This is important when establishing honest connection and understanding. The difference is, when it comes from a truly confident person (rather than a vulnerable person) there is no room for attack or abuse.

Back to Self-Honesty

Regardless of how humans came to be, whether that is from millions of years of evolution, walking out of the Garden of Eden, or being put here by aliens, we are born to learn about our world, but more specifically, learn who we honestly are. To do this, we have to do something we are not used to doing. We have to get radically self-honest and practice the art of honestly listening while in a blame-free mindset.

When we are looking to exit our inherited victim mindset, we don't have to point our finger at any party. The goal is not to find fault but to entertain the possibility that we contributed to the outcome, regardless of how insignificant that might seem. That contribution will be linked to our self-honesty. Like the person who wants to kill themselves and sees the car coming but closes their eyes instead of moving out of the way. It is the same as the person who desperately wished for something to happen to get them out of a difficult situation. Crossing your fingers. Praying to your God or a guardian angel to intervene so you didn't have to face your phobia and talk in public. Sometimes the help arrives in a way we don't consciously want, but that doesn't negate the fact we had something to contribute. Just like Derek Redmond's experience at the 1992 Olympics. He got more than he imagined in a way he could never have imagined.

We are often happy to take credit for the part we played in an experience when we like the result. But the blame fingers are quickly unholstered if we perceive something as unhelpful, hurtful, bad, negative, wrong, a mistake, or a failure. It is like taking credit for winning the lottery because you bought a ticket and chose numbers related to your family birthdays. But then thinking it is unfair, unlucky, bad, and wrong if you lost all your money investing it in your brother's new tech startup. In reality, we put the same effort into co-creating every experience we have. It is our black-and-white thinking while in our victim mindset that shuts out this wisdom.

Gaining access to our self-honesty helps us make sense of the world. For example, there are so many people walking around feeling deeply unhappy, angry, fearful, and lost. Suicide is on the increase all around the world. Many are successful in their attempts, while many are not. Isn't it possible that many more people are *unconsciously* acting this out? Just like the people with a broken heart who suddenly die of a mysterious and fatal illness as the thought of living without their partner is too much to bear. Or people like my father who died six months after he retired because his reason for living was gone. There are so many people wishing harm, revenge, and pain onto themselves and others. Could this influence what happens in their life? Maybe similar experiences would show up in their life to mirror back their honest emotional state rather than the fake one they show to the world.

I offered this to my client John who came to me with a label of Parkinson's disease. I said, when we look at what your body is doing, it is shaking with anger. Understandably, at first, he balked at the idea. He had bought into the label and diagnosis so no other possibilities existed, especially any to do with the idea his body was helping him. As he became more self-honest, he agreed that his symptoms did get more extreme the more rage he felt. His extreme physical and mental condition was matched by the extreme number of blame- and victim-based stories he had in his arsenal. Everyone was to blame for why his life worked out the way it did. He was unknowingly broadcasting his honest emotional state (anger, rage, hatred) even when he thought he had done a good job hiding it from himself and others. And distance is not a limiting factor when it comes to projecting our honest state of being.

When we start to fathom the interconnectedness of everything via energy, frequency, and vibration, people all around the globe will pick up on our self-honest state. Hence, why moms, twins, or people we are close to reach out when they feel a disturbance in the force, as Luke Skywalker might say.

John had a lightbulb moment. He shared a story with me that happened twenty years before. It was the catalyst for why he started seeking help for his anger issues. Something had infuriated him, and as a way of burning off the anger he stormed out of the house for a walk. After about thirty minutes he caught the eye of someone across the busy road. Within seconds they were in each other's face having an aggressive confrontation. John's new realization was, he had looked into the eyes of many people in that half an hour, but the one person who matched the frequency of his rage was the one who responded.

People who believe in karma—or the repackaged modern-day version, the law of attraction—would advocate that this is a perfect example to illustrate how they work. Good attracts good, bad attracts bad. They would consider a fight in the middle of Fifth Avenue, NYC, as bad. However, this is not the case. When blame isn't part of the equation, something very different materializes. John was like a magnet, tuned at a frequency that would pull in the same level of rage like an iron filing. They were both mirroring each other's self-honesty. Not to punish them, but to give them an opportunity to self-reflect and get honest so they could ultimately heal.

John's contribution to this extreme experience was his anger, rage, and hatred for people in his life (and himself). But where did this originate? It came from his blame addiction, but where did that come from? The reality is: our emotional state and contribution to our extremely painful experiences could be centuries in the making.

Traditional Influence

Could creating, accepting, and passing on certain traditions or creation myths be our contribution to what we co-create as an individual and as a species? What if someone accepts the tradition that women are inferior or sexual objects? It wasn't until the second half of the twentieth century that marital rape was even considered a legal issue. Prior to that, as stated by Sir Matthew Hale, an influential English judge in the seventeenth century, "The husband cannot be guilty of a rape committed by himself upon his lawful wife…" This sentiment is mirrored all around the world as some husbands have the legal right to discipline their wife and children with physical force.

What if a creation myth is built on a foundation of revenge, murder, or infanticide…or if it is said you are born into sin? Could this become an unconscious influence in what we bring into reality? Could having genitalia mutilated as a baby through circumcision be a tradition that contributes to the amount of self-blame (self-hatred) and sexual issues we have? Could it confirm there is something wrong with us? It is fair to say that we are unaware of most of what influences our perception and decisions and the experiences they lead to.

What I have come to realize is that we were born with a foundation saturated in blame addiction, victimhood, and fear, and this is unknowingly nurtured from day one by others who are unaware they inherited the same foundational elements. This is the main contributing factor that overrides all others.

It was a game changer for me to realize that all the while I accepted certain passed traditions and concepts, I was feeding my blame addiction. My mind, body, and life would then reflect and resemble that of a powerless victim. I would believe their underlying message and be convinced I either had no contribution to my life or that certain experiences weren't helping me. Neither of which are true. As I have demonstrated many times throughout this book, when we train our perception muscle, we have access to more information, awareness, and wisdom. It is a process that opens the doors of possibility. The more that opened, the more I discovered who I honestly was. The more comfortable I got at being self-honest, the better I got at connecting the dots. I could see how certain experiences materialized and why they were more extreme than previous ones. My mind, body, and life would then reflect and resemble that of a confident leader of my life.

The idea that we are contributing to every experience in our life can be a confusing and triggering part of my philosophy. This was highlighted during a leadership program I was running in South Africa. One of the participants stopped me and said, "So you don't think rape is bad!" I had been here many times, as jumping to the most extreme abuse we can think of is where people often go when I talk about this subject. It is important to address these extreme instances, but if that is where we focus, we won't see the benefits of applying this philosophy to everyday situations. We need to practice on the low-level events so we don't co-create the extremely painful ones.

With that said, I assured the room, if they were to ask me a different question, we would all be on the same page. If they asked, "Do I want to live in a world where rape exists?" the answer is categorically no. What I am offering is a new way that it can be stopped. Because as far as I can see, the one we have been putting into practice is only seeing rape become more prevalent. The model of victimizing the victim and bullying the bully hoping it will stop is creating more blame, victims, anger, and fear, which all equal more abuse. We can only build so many prisons before our planet becomes one big prison.

Just because we don't label an incident as bad, negative, or wrong doesn't mean we view it as good, positive, or right.

Healing comes as we exit this blame-based dichotomous mindset. I am also not advocating we scrap the legal system as I have been accused. My goal is to help people out of the Victim Cycle so they co-create fewer instances that see them having to enter a courtroom in the first place.

To understand how extreme events happen, we have to consider some of the smaller situations that inevitably preceded the big one. Before every major traumatic event, there were minor incidents where the same feelings came up at lower decibels. But we ignored those smaller situations and things escalated. This can happen over a day, week, year, or decade. But it can also happen over thousands of years.

To help the South African group, I used a client example to illustrate a point. Chloe came to me after a violent attack that happened while she was out on a run in the middle of the day. She decided to run around the park one more time before she went home. And during this final loop, she was mugged at knifepoint.

There are two main types of responses people might commonly have to a story like Chloe's. The first would be to sympathize, tell her it wasn't her fault, and condemn her attacker as pure evil. The second would be to smother her in positive self-help platitudes and encourage her to let it go, forgive and forget, and move on. Both of these reactions are unknowingly based in blame. This might help Chloe push the painful feelings under the rug for a while, but it doesn't help her heal, which would prevent similar experiences in the future. These approaches rest on the narrative that Chloe is an innocent victim and not only does she have nothing to contribute to the experience, but she also has nothing to gain. It keeps her in a constant state of fear (anxiety) to the point that she doesn't want to go out of her house.

Chloe had received sympathy and a growing list of platitudes. Under the brave exterior, fear was growing. Her self-blame was being well fed. She was doing a good job of beating herself up for not going home when she should have. "Why did I run one more lap?" she constantly asked herself.

I mentioned that when it comes to the bigger picture of healing, one of the main reasons we co-create anything is to become aware of our honest emotional state.

Full of empathy for her experience, I asked, "How did you feel during the attack?"

"Afraid and alone," she said in a small voice.

I commented that I was sure, leading up to this attack, there would have been other less dramatic events that left her feeling *afraid* and *alone*. After a moment of quiet, she confirmed this to be true. She also later confessed that she only took up running recently to cope with the stress of these very instances. Feeling afraid and alone had been something she had been dealing with all her life. She used sex and drugs from a young age to feel confident, popular, and loved.

I made sure the South African group recognized that Chloe didn't want to be *mugged*. This is an important part of the co-creation process. She just needed an incrementally more extreme experience to bring out her honest and underlying emotional state. And for her, this experience was it. For another person, like a professional MMA fighter or a Navy SEAL, being mugged in this way wouldn't have been extreme enough to elicit the same feelings. They might have needed to break a leg and fall down a ditch during their run to feel afraid and alone.

One of the participants said to me, "So what you're saying is that if we are not in the Victim Cycle as you say, the chances of us experiencing these extreme situations diminish?" And that is it. As we recover from our blame addiction, fear, anger, and the need for revenge or abuse of any type have no kindling. There is nothing to ignite all these blame-based emotions. As this is replicated in a society, the desire to abuse anyone disappears.

There is a different cycle we can partake in. As we make our way around the Self-Healing Cycle, the more healthy, harmonious, and effortless our life becomes.

New Cycle

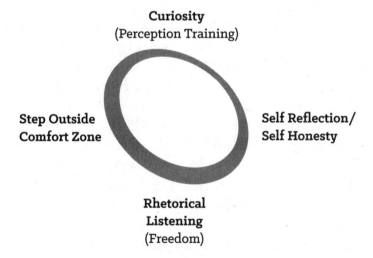

Curiosity
(Perception Training)

Step Outside
Comfort Zone

Self Reflection/
Self Honesty

Rhetorical
Listening
(Freedom)

The more I recovered from my blame addiction, the more I came to understand how self-healing and life are designed to be effortless. I found myself in a very different cycle than the victim one I had become accustomed to. My curiosity to question what I had accepted as true led me to train my perception muscle. No longer happy to see the world in black and white, I sought out the color that came with finding other possibilities in how I contributed to all my experiences. As I did, I naturally became less angry, fearful, shameful, guilty, and regretful. It provided the space and incentive to self-reflect and get honest with myself. It would help me become aware of where I was playing the Blame Game and seeking control. I would then naturally want to grow and expand, which would take me outside my comfort zone.

As each cycle completed, I became more and more aware how all roads led back to me, and my dishonesty had been fueling so much of the fear, anger, shame, guilt, regret, and pain in my life. I realized more than ever that my blame addiction was the foundation of all other addictions. The reason we need substances and habitual behaviors is because we are looking for a way to numb us from our mental and emotional pain. But where did this pain ultimately come from? From blaming ourselves, parents, siblings, society, governments, corporations, teachers, bosses, and partners for doing something bad, negative, and wrong.

As justifiable as this blame feels considering all the corruption and abuse that goes on in the world, I started to really question what created all this in the first place. It is us spinning around in the Victim Cycle where we keep controlling, accepting, and being dishonest. It just leads to more and more extreme pain to encourage us to enter the Self-Healing Cycle. As we recover from our addiction to playing the Blame Game, we pass on a very different foundation for future generations to build on.

Soon a new sense of mental, emotional, and physical freedom enveloped me as I made my way around this new self-perpetuating cycle. The less mental and emotional pain I had, the less physical pain I experienced. Less physical pain meant less mental and emotional pain. My newfound fearlessness, confidence, and freedom would once again take me out of my comfort zone. I wanted more out of life. I wanted to help more people experience the effortlessness and freedom that I knew was available to everyone.

One of the practical ways to notice if you are honestly healing and changing is to keep a note of how effortless your life is becoming. As blame leaves your system, there is less pain and conflict. Life just seems to get easier. More synchronicities happen. To aid the change process, you have to collect your own bank of evidence.

To do this, we have to practice something else we are not used to doing: noticing what is different as opposed to what is the same.

Difference Diary

To help my clients stay in the Self-Healing Cycle, I suggest they start writing a Difference Diary. I didn't realize I was doing this when I started writing *The Blame Game* over the last decade. Unknowingly, I was documenting all the changes, synchronicities, and differences in my life (and my clients') during my own self-discovery adventure. If I wasn't writing down my changes and amazing "coincidences," I was discussing them with friends and family. The rest of the time I was explaining how those differences and experiences came about to clients. It was while working with one client, Laura, that I realized how useful it could be for others to do the same.

Laura and her mother always seemed to butt heads. Laura felt judged (blamed) by her mother at every turn—from her appearance, to her career choices, to her sexual identity. She had spent over twenty-five years "working on herself," but the tension remained whenever she spent time with her mom.

I started working with Laura once per week and after three weeks she told me nothing had changed in her life. It happens from time to time because we get so used to putting on the same T-shirt every morning that reads, "Same shit, different day!" Laura had a whole wardrobe full of them. At the beginning of every session, she would tell me why her way of thinking was right and mine was wrong, even though after thinking the "right" way, she was nearing financial, mental, and physical bankruptcy.

When I asked Laura what was different during the previous week, she would reply before I even finished asking the question, "Nothing!" Her answer was a little too quick to be the whole truth. Enquiring about whether she had written in the Difference Diary was met with, "There was no point; I had nothing to put in it." In this situation I go into interviewer mode. In order to open Laura's mind so she could look past her cognitive bias, I start grilling her about every single detail of her week, including how she ate, drank, slept, exercised, and socialized. I drilled into every interaction she had. How work, home, and her hobbies were going. What she watched on TV, listened to on Spotify. Any "coincidences" that occurred.

Seemingly random purchases, decisions, or creative pursuits. No stone was left unturned.

After a full breakdown, we uncovered changes she had overlooked. Lo and behold, from that point forward we always found differences. She had also been looking for "big" changes. Occasionally saying, "Nothing significant changed this week." Not realizing this was another way of confirming her cognitive bias. All the while we have our blame blinkers on, we aren't aware of the bigger picture impact of the seemingly small changes in our lives. This is why having—and using—a Difference Diary is so important.

I did the same with a couple who told me that nothing had changed after our first session. They disappointingly told me they were still arguing. I asked them how long it took for them to resolve their fights. On reflection, it was a shocking realization to acknowledge that it only took minutes whereas previously it could be hours or even days before any normality resumed. They focused on the same (the fight), not the difference (how long it took to become friends again).

With one foot out of the Victim Cycle, Laura acknowledged that she actually experienced quite a significant difference. One that during our first session she assured me would never happen. Her relationship with her mother started to change. Her mother greeted her by asking how she was. This was a big difference, Laura said, because she was used to being met with criticism or what she felt like were passive-aggressive jabs such as, "Oh, you've cut your hair," or "Have you put on weight?" As the self-honesty door opened, Laura also mentioned her partner commented on how different her mother had been to them the last time they got together, asking how they were doing and being genuinely interested in what they had to say.

Laura had an agenda. Her mother was the biggest enemy in her life. She had decades of victim-based stories proving this to be the truth and nothing but the truth. Focusing on any difference would oppose her hardened victim story. I suggested she put more effort into jotting down any difference she noticed.

Looking for clarification, she said, "You mean like a gratitude journal?"

She told me that one of the reasons she hadn't given the Difference Diary much attention, was because she had been writing one of those for the last four years. It opened up a long discussion around how this practice was keeping her in a victim mindset. Forcing gratitude or any emotion that is perceived as positive feels great. But what does this practice ultimately teach us? To again be fake positive and divide our experiences into rigid camps of good and bad. If we are not naturally feeling grateful, then it teaches us to be dishonest. There is a difference between forcing ourselves to be grateful and finding ourselves feeling grateful as a by-product of new awareness. I mentioned how I am in a constant state of awe at how beautifully orchestrated life is to give me ever more extreme opportunities to find out who I honestly am. But I have never forced myself to be grateful or done any gratitude journaling to get there.

A month of writing her Difference Diary in a way that didn't class things as positive or negative helped Laura become more aware of how significantly her perceptions and life were shifting.

What I'm advocating is not a typical journaling exercise where we write down our feelings. By focusing on what's different every day, we can increase our awareness and flex our perception muscles. We can train ourselves to see in color. And with greater awareness comes motivation to continue on the journey. We naturally do this every time we buy a new phone or car. We might not commonly write anything down, but we do notice what is different. It helps us keep it or return it.

Noticing what is different is an invaluable part of the honesty healing journey. Even if you open up the diary and write nothing down, the fact you entered that space is enough. The next time you hear yourself say, "Nothing ever works out for me," "I always have bad luck," or "Same shit, different day!" You will pause and realize this is a lie. You can then look back over the diary and see all the changes that have occurred. Because most of my clients experience a profound shift in their lives, often in short periods of time, they can forget what life was like before. They forget how hard life was and want more of the changes they are experiencing. Having a resource to remind us how far we have come provides the reality check we sometimes need.

Effortless living needs effort before it becomes effortless. At this stage of our evolution, we are making lying and being a victim effortless. When we put effort into self-reflecting, being self-honest, rhetorically listening and noticing differences, life just gets easier. Things just fall into place. People want to help you as much as you want to help them. There is a learning curve to this, and it can be steep, but it doesn't have to be.

Attaining profound feelings of freedom and liberation can be effortless. Especially when you experience other people change as you honestly heal. Seeing your ecosystem effortlessly change—and maintain that change with no control or fake positivity—is a clear reflection that you have honestly healed.

The Ripple Effect

I often get asked to help babies or children. My response to the parent is normally the same: "I will help them by helping you first." Amira was one such mother who was distraught at hearing the news her young girl had kidney disease. Her daughter had been on antibiotics for the majority of her three years of life and was destined to be on them for many more years.

A week after taking Amira through the honest healing process, I received a very emotional voice message detailing how the doctor said the impossible had happened. The disease was gone. Amira said in her message, "It is amazing that such a small change in me can have such a dramatic effect on my daughter!" Amira's anger was not only creating inflammation in her own body but it was emanating for the whole family to pick up on. They all received it and reacted differently. Her husband walked on eggshells shutting himself away, while her daughter, not having the emotional maturity or ability to run away, took on the anger as it matched what she had inherited.

Amira's daughter was acting like a mirror, reflecting back her unhappiness and frustration. As Amira healed, her daughter felt it and relaxed mentally and physically. Because her daughter didn't understand or accept the label of "kidney disease," she now had the perfect environment to rejuvenate.

Eliana was one of my very first clients. It was her story that hit me like a blow from Thor's hammer. It woke me up to what is possible when we honestly heal. I initially treated

Eliana's husband for a few labels, including stress, anxiety, and a slipped disk. Following a few successful sessions, he eagerly arranged for Eliana to see me, as she had similar complaints. It was her answer to my first question—"How can I help you?"—that opened my eyes. "Well the funny thing is," she said, "since you have been helping my husband, my two-year chronic back pain has completely gone." She actually wanted help with her confusion, as she couldn't understand how this was possible. Wide-eyed, she asked, "What happened?"

During our session, Eliana confessed she saw herself as a failure in the relationship. Nothing she did to ease her husband's stress and physical pain worked. The fact is, she felt responsible for her husband's happiness and well-being. She reasoned, "That is the role of a good wife." Because of all the self-blame, she didn't realize how her increasingly painful and chronic back pain was benefitting her and asking her to address something deeper. It is no different to how a plant wilts and discolors to bring attention to itself.

As her husband's pain became more severe, he became more irritable and short-tempered. His angry outbursts were often directed toward her. Unconsciously she worked out that the more pain she exhibited, the less blame and anger she received—more pain equaled more sympathy. She was using her victimhood to her advantage. It worked for a while until even this strategy couldn't buffer the blame and anger. In a moment of self-honesty, Eliana admitted, to counter this she would exaggerate the pain or even fake it altogether in order to placate her husband. As much as this worked in one way, it induced a lot of guilt and shame due to her dishonesty, which created more stress and more back pain.

She was very much in the Victim Cycle. She had been waiting for her husband to change. Like many people, she felt responsibility for how others feel. She did it with her family and friends—not realizing this energetically bound them, meaning she could experience similar (phantom) psychological and physiological stressors. I explained the principle outlined in chapter 1: that whatever we do isn't what ultimately impacts another person's feelings or behavior. It is whatever fuels *their* perception of what we did or said that results in their emotional response and behavior.

My aim was to really help Eliana understand that the more self-honest (and selfish) we are to heal ourselves, the more it paradoxically helps other people change. Pushing this point felt important, as she expressed how powerless she felt when she wanted to help her husband. Her back pain disappeared because her husband's blame towards her subsided. She could relax, and didn't need her back pain to help her out of a difficult situation anymore. As much as this was a great example to explain how blame works and how our bodies are always helping us in weird and wonderful ways, she would also benefit from learning how to recover from her blame addiction. This would minimize the need to evoke emotionally and physically painful victim experiences in the future to experience joy and freedom.

Anger, disappointment, frustration, guilt, shame, and regret are all indicators we are in a state of blame. In the same way, referring to something as bad, negative, wrong, a mistake, or failure are all barometers indicating we are swirling around in the Victim Cycle. They are all moments to encourage us to self-reflect and listen to our mind and body.

You Are One of the Crazy Ones

If you have gotten this far, then you are most definitely one of the crazy ones cited in Steve Jobs' famous quote. The quote is worth repeating here:

> Here's to the crazy ones. The misfits. The rebels. The troublemakers. The round pegs in the square holes. The ones who see things differently. They're not fond of rules. And they have no respect for the status quo. You can quote them, disagree with them, glorify or vilify them. But the only thing you can't do is ignore them. Because they change things. They push the human race forward. And while some may see them as the crazy ones, we see genius. Because the people who are crazy enough to think they can change the world are the ones who do.

I realized more than ever after reading this quote that I am one of the crazy ones. At the start, my clients don't realize they are also the same. They don't realize they are changing the world. They don't initially realize they are doing so in the most profound and impactful way possible...by honestly healing themselves from a blame addiction they never knew they had.

My mission is to change the course of history. Not because I think we are going the wrong way, but because I can feel there is a different way. One that the world has long forgotten. A world where blame, fear, control, and being a victim isn't our driving force.

The end result of blame is conflict, abuse, division, and finally separation. All aspects of our world are reflecting back the fact we are in the advanced state of our addiction to playing the Blame Game. It is why we have an abundance of fear, pain, abuse, hatred, and need for revenge in our world. And why we think it is 'normal' to have arguments with our partners, friends and family members. It isn't. All screaming matches are extreme indicators that you are firmly in the Victim Cycle. This is why most of our relationships end in separation, not because of incompatibility but because of excessive blame and how we compete for the best victim story.

Blame is a human construct. It isn't found anywhere else in nature. It is why when nature is left to do what nature is designed to do, it rejuvenates and regenerates very quickly after it experiences trauma. Humans have found it incredibly difficult to honestly heal up till now because we have been swimming in blame like a fish in water. It feels so natural and normal it has become interwoven into the very fabric of our reality and vocabulary. There has been little desire to change it. And when we have, we only had control-and-conquer tools, techniques, and modalities at our disposal. We have also gotten used to giving our power over to others, which is why I am not looking for your trust, faith, or hope. I want you to establish your own deep knowing, which comes from your personal experimentation and evidence.

More than ever in our history, it is time to question what we have accepted as truth so we can think and live differently. I am not offering a new version of truth; I am just offering an alternative way of looking at life. And I have redefined Murphy's Law to help you remember the simplicity of what I am ultimately offering: anything you think has gone wrong is here to help you discover who you honestly are.

It is a simple interpretation of a very complex existence. But paradoxically, it is this simplicity that helps me understand the complexity. I am now aware that our world works in weird and wonderful ways, all with one purpose. A purpose we all share. To help us find out who we honestly are so we can co-create a life based on that person, and not the fake one we present to the world. All so we can reach levels of potential, freedom, and joy we didn't realize were possible.

About the Author

Denis Liam Murphy is a high-performance coach, visionary thinker, and founding partner of RoundTable Global, an internationally recognized learning and development company that helps create high-performance leaders and corporate cultural change. He is also the founding partner of BeyondBamboo, a company offering planet conscious products, procurement, and consultancy services to individuals and organizations all over the world.

Murphy offers a truly unique and unparalleled personal development and healing experience by specializing in helping people recover from a blame addiction they didn't know they had. To do this, he combines over fifteen years of entrepreneurial experience with extensive worldwide travel and cultural exposure. After thousands of hours working with clients, Murphy has gained an in-depth knowledge of human behavior, healing, and energy medicine to help people reach new levels of honesty, happiness, success, and optimal performance in timeframes that are often considered impossible.